ULTIMATE YOGA GUIDE FOR HEART HEALTH

Unlocking the Healing Power of Yoga: A Comprehensive Guide with Pictorial Postures and Heart-Healthy Diets for Strengthening Your Heart, Soothing Your Mind, and Elevating Your Well-Being.

BY

DR. KAMA KAMZY

Introduction: Welcome To a Heart-Healthy Journey

A woman named Maya lived in the bustling city of Calmington, where the speed of life frequently resembled the quick beats of the heart. Maya was no stranger to the challenges of a frenetic profession, combining long hours at a high-stress job with day-to-day duties. She had no idea her heart was speaking its yearning for change as she navigated her hectic daily.

Maya's life took an unexpected turn one beautiful autumn morning. It began off like any other day, dashing between meetings and deadlines. But as the hours passed, a terrifying tightness grabbed her chest—a pressure that refused to go away. She shook it aside, blaming it on the constant tension she had gotten accustomed to.

When the sensation lingered throughout the evening, she realized she couldn't ignore it any longer. Unease gnawed at her, forcing her to seek assistance. She made her way to the neighborhood health center with reluctance.

Her heart hammered in time with her steps as she entered the clinic. She had no idea that this was the first step in her heart-healthy path. I greeted her with a kind grin. He listened intently as she detailed her symptoms, interrogating her about her lifestyle and everyday stresses.

Maya, like many of us, had been lost in the turmoil of life, ignoring the very center of her being—her heart. I carefully discussed the significance of heart health and the role that stress may play in its degradation, using my wealth of knowledge and compassion.

Maya felt a spark of insight after that chat. She understood her heart was more than simply a necessary organ; it was also a sign of her happiness, fortitude, and potential for joy. Maya set out on a heart-healthy quest, determined to change her life.

Dr. Kamzy introduced her to the transformational power of yoga, an ancient discipline that not only strengthens but also heals the body and spirit. Yoga became Maya's refuge, an oasis of peace in the midst of mayhem. She felt the tightness in her body dissolve with each asana, allowing her fresh power and flexibility.

However, yoga was only one element of the puzzle. Maya also discovered the value of mindful eating, embracing a heart-healthy diet. She realized that the food she ate was more than simply fuel; it was medication for her heart and soul.

Maya's heart underwent an amazing change as the weeks evolved into months. The tension in her chest began to dissipate, replaced with a sensation of lightness and vibrancy. She became more resilient in the face of stress, and her heartbeats seemed to echo a soothing tune.

Maya's heart-healthy journey not only changed her life, but it also affected the lives of others around her. Friends and family watched her improvement and were motivated to follow in her footsteps to better heart health. A community of people devoted to cultivating their hearts and souls began to thrive in the heart of Calmington.

This book, **"Ultimate Yoga Guide for Heart Health"** is an invitation—a warm welcome to join Maya on her heart-healthy journey. These pages include Dr. Kamzy's knowledge, the transformational force of yoga, and the nourishment of heart-healthy eating. Most significantly, you'll discover your own heart's capacity for resiliency, vigor, and long-term well-being.

So, while we go through the chapters ahead, keep in mind that your heart is more than simply an organ—it's the compass of your existence. Welcome to a heart-healthy journey where transformation is on the horizon and your heart's aspirations are respected.

Chapter 1: Understanding Yoga and Heart Health

Key Facts and a Quick Overview
Introduction:

Yoga, an ancient Indian discipline, has crossed generations and cultures to become a global phenomenon. Yoga is more than just physical postures and stretches; it is a comprehensive approach to well-being that supports not just the body but also the mind and spirit. Yoga has had a significant impact on heart health, providing a natural and comprehensive technique to enhance cardiovascular well-being. In this quick overview, we'll look at some essential facts concerning the relationship between yoga and heart health.

- The Holistic Approach of Yoga

Yoga is a philosophy that seeks harmony between the self and the universe as a whole, not only exercise. Its holistic approach highlights the interdependence of the body, mind, and spirit. When it comes to heart health, this involves addressing not only physical fitness but also mental and emotional well-being, both of which play important roles in heart health.

- Stress Management and Heart Health

Stress reduction is one of the most important ways yoga benefits heart health. Chronic stress has long been recognized as a risk factor for heart disease. Relaxation practices in yoga, such as deep breathing and meditation, have been demonstrated to lower stress hormones, drop blood pressure, and produce a sense of calm—a boon to the heart in today's fast-paced world.

- Cardiovascular Advantages of Physical Asanas

Yoga incorporates a diverse variety of physical postures or asanas, ranging from simple stretches to more rigorous exercises. These asanas help increase circulation, flexibility, and heart muscle strength. Backbends and inversions, for example, can have special benefits for heart health.

- Heart Rate Control and Mindful Breathing

Pranayama, or yogic breathing, focuses on conscious and regulated inhaling and exhalation. Individuals can alter their heart rate variability with pranayama practices, creating a healthy balance between the sympathetic and parasympathetic neural systems. This, in turn, has the potential to improve heart health.

- Yoga's Role in Weight Loss

Maintaining a healthy weight is critical for cardiovascular health. Yoga, when paired with a healthy diet, can help with weight loss by raising consciousness about eating patterns and encouraging physical exercise.

- Heart Health and Emotional Resilience

The heart is directly affected by emotions. Yoga promotes emotional resilience by teaching people how to deal with stress, anxiety, and negative emotions. Mindfulness and meditation can help practitioners achieve emotional well-being, which improves the heart.

We'll discover the subtle ways in which yoga practices might promote cardiovascular fitness as we go deeper into this investigation of yoga and heart health. This journey provides insights and resources to empower you on your way to a healthy heart, from learning the science behind yoga's influence on the heart to discovering practical yoga sequences geared to heart health.

The Heart: The Powerhouse of Your Happiness

The heart, a wonderful organ, is sometimes portrayed as a symbol of love, although its significance extends well beyond romantic problems. It is the genuine powerhouse of life, the guardian of our well-being, and the conductor of our joy.

We often fail to pause and reflect on the tremendous significance our hearts play in a world filled with the hustle and bustle of daily life. It is more than simply a pump that pumps blood; it is the protector of our existence. Let us untangle the deep relationship between our emotional well-being and the physical organ lying between our chests as we begin on this journey to comprehend the heart as the powerhouse of happiness.

A Symbiotic Relationship Between the Heart and Emotions

We've all felt it: the quickening of the heart in times of excitement, the sinking sensation in the chest in times of grief, and the fluttering sensation in times of love. These bodily feelings are not random; they are the heart's method of communicating with us.

The heart and emotions are inextricably linked. Psychophysiology research has revealed that the heart and brain constantly exchange information. The heart-brain link, a communication network, is critical in controlling our emotional reactions.

Poets and philosophers have lauded the heart as the seat of emotions for generations. Science is now providing evidence to back up this claim. The heart is home to a network of neurons and chemicals that can affect our emotional state. In essence, your heart influences how you feel. It is actively influencing your emotions rather than simply responding to them.

The Heart and Happiness Science

To understand how the heart affects our happiness, we must go to science. The thymus gland, a little pinecone-shaped gland situated beneath the breastbone, lies at the heart of this link. This gland has been related to the generation of T lymphocytes, a kind of white blood cell that plays an important role in immunological function.

Recent study has found that the thymus gland is more than just a component in our immune system; it also plays an important role in our mental well-being. It serves as a link between our physical and mental wellness.

The thymus gland secretes hormones that improve our immune system and promote general well-being when we feel pleasant emotions such as love, joy, or appreciation. In essence, the emotions we nurture have a direct influence on the heart's health and lifespan.

The Resilience of the Heart: A Key to Happiness

The heart is a source of resilience as well as an emotional gauge. It has an amazing capacity to adapt to difficult situations. When we are confronted with hardship, our hearts respond by generating stress hormones. While chronic stress can be harmful to the heart, moderate, short-term stress can actually strengthen it.

Consider it a cardiovascular exercise. Lifting weights builds your muscles, and dealing with life's hardships in moderation strengthens your heart. It becomes more robust, more able to deal with life's ups and downs, and hence contributes to your overall happiness.

Yoga as a Route to Heart-Centered Happiness

In our journey to understand the function of the heart in happiness, we come upon a great ally: yoga. This ancient practice, which includes physical postures, breath control, and meditation, provides a profound internal trip—a voyage to the center of our pleasure.

Yoga, which is typically lauded for its physical advantages, is also beneficial to the heart. When performed attentively, physical asanas boost cardiovascular health by increasing circulation, lowering blood pressure, and general heart function.

However, yoga extends beyond the physical. It invites us to journey across our emotional landscapes. We acquire insights into our emotional responses via mindfulness and meditation, learning to negotiate stress, anxiety, and negativity with grace.

One of the pillars of yoga is the practice of appreciation and love—qualities that are inextricably tied to the health of the heart. We boost the heart's resiliency and increase our overall happiness by fostering these feelings.

The Influence of Heart-Centered Living

As we go through life, keep in mind that our hearts aren't just bystanders in the big scheme of things. They are the orchestrators, directors, and architects of our enjoyment. Our hearts are the well-being engines that shape our emotional landscapes and influence our physical health.

Accept the heart-centered way of living. Develop love, appreciation, and resilience. Explore the transforming practice of yoga, and you'll discover that happiness isn't just a distant fantasy, but just a heartbeat away. The heart, your constant partner on this trip, is ready to lead you to a life of happiness, energy, and long-term well-being.

The Science of Yoga and Heart Health

Yoga, an ancient practice that unites the mind, body, and spirit, has recently earned widespread attention for its significant influence on heart health. While yoga has long been lauded for its mental and physical advantages, a closer look at its scientific foundations reveals a strong link between yoga and heart health.

1. *Stress Reduction as a Heart-Healthy Foundation*

Stress, an ever-present companion in modern life, is crucial to cardiovascular health. Chronic stress causes the production of hormones such as cortisol and adrenaline, which raises blood pressure and contributes to inflammation, which is a risk factor for heart disease.

Yoga, with its emphasis on relaxation and mindfulness, is an effective stress reliever. Regular yoga practice has been demonstrated in scientific research to reduce the production of stress hormones, lower blood pressure, and enhance relaxation responses in the body. This, in turn, benefits heart health by lowering cardiovascular system wear and strain.

2. *Improved Cardiac Function: The Physical Asanas of Yoga*

The physical part of yoga, known as asanas or poses, has enormous promise for improving heart health. Yoga asanas range from simple stretches to rigorous positions, and each improves circulation and cardiovascular function.

According to research, yoga asanas can increase blood flow, cardiac muscle strength, and overall heart function. Downward-Facing Dog, Cobra, and Bridge Pose are especially good for heart health because they stimulate the chest and upper body muscles, boosting heart strength and flexibility.

3. *Heart Rate Variability and Mindful Breathing*

Breath is an essential component of yoga practice, and it has a significant impact on heart health. Pranayama, or yogic breathing methods, emphasize regulated and aware intake and exhalation. These approaches not only relax the mind but also have an effect on the heart.

According to research, pranayama techniques help modulate heart rate variability (HRV), a key indicator of cardiac health. HRV is a measure of the time difference between successive heartbeats and is linked to stress resilience. Yoga promotes heart health by improving HRV and establishing a healthy autonomic nervous system response.

4. *Inflammation Reduction: Yoga's Anti-Inflammatory Effects*

Chronic inflammation is a major cause of heart disease. Yoga has been found to lower inflammatory indicators such as C-reactive protein (CRP) and interleukin-6 (IL-6). This anti-inflammatory action is very beneficial in the prevention and treatment of heart disease.

5. *Emotional well-being and cardiovascular health*

Emotions, which are frequently seen as the domain of the heart, have a significant influence on cardiovascular health. Chronic stress, anxiety, and depression are all established risk factors for heart disease.

Yoga, with its emphasis on emotional resilience and mindfulness, assists people in navigating these emotions gracefully. Yoga promotes emotional well-being by encouraging meditation and the cultivation of pleasant feelings such as appreciation and compassion.

6. *Changes in Lifestyle and Behavior*

Yoga is more than simply a set of physical postures; it is a way of life that promotes overall well-being. Adopting a heart-healthy lifestyle is part of this. Yoga practitioners frequently become more conscious of their eating habits, physical exercise, and general health.

Yoga helps to better heart health outcomes and a lower risk of heart disease by encouraging these favorable lifestyle modifications.

Finally, the science of yoga and heart health is an enthralling investigation into the mind-body relationship. It demonstrates how this ancient practice, which is based on mindfulness and self-care, may have a significant influence on the cardiovascular system. Yoga provides a comprehensive approach to heart health that integrates ancient wisdom with current science, thereby developing a stronger, happier heart.

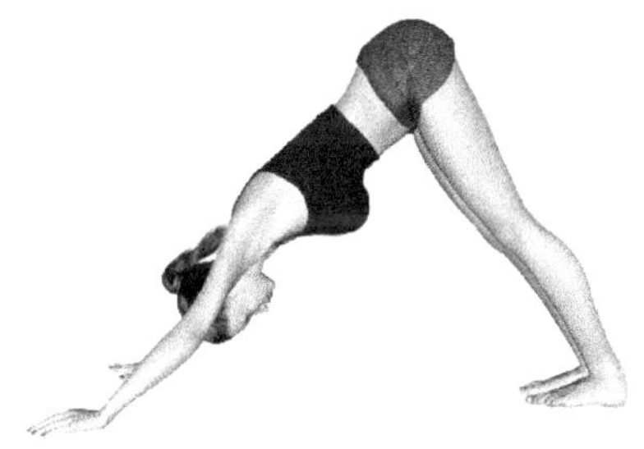

Downward-Facing Dog Position

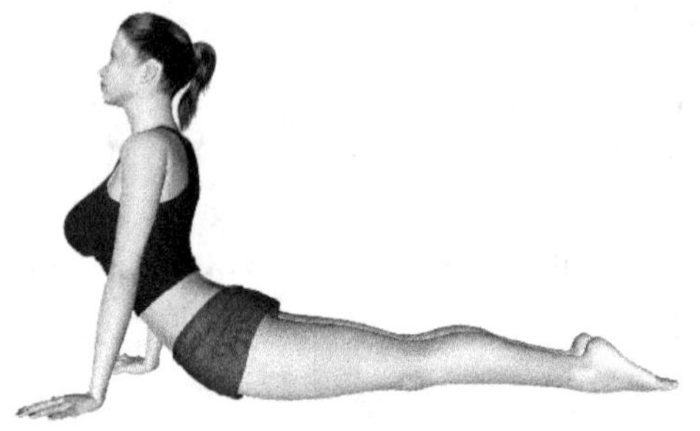

Cobra Position

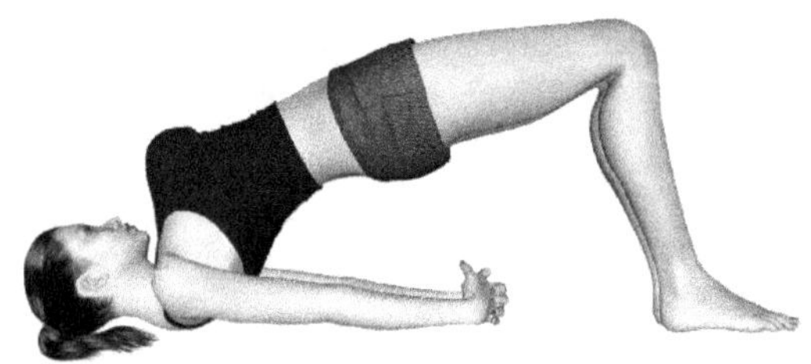

Bridge Pose Position

The Holistic Approach of Yoga to Cardiovascular Wellness

The importance of cardiovascular fitness cannot be stressed in our fast-paced society, when stress, sedentary lifestyles, and bad food habits have become the norm. Heart disease, the leading cause of death worldwide, necessitates a comprehensive and integrated strategy to prevention and care. Enter yoga, a centuries-old practice that has emerged as an effective tool in the pursuit of cardiovascular health.

Yoga's Transformative Power

Meet another of my patients. Sarah is a lady in her mid-forties who, like many in our modern culture, found herself imprisoned in the midst of a high-stress profession and a sedentary lifestyle. Her frantic schedule left little time for exercise or self-care, and stress became an unpleasant companion. Sarah had a palpitation one fateful day, which sent shockwaves of dread through her body.

She sought medical guidance from me after being terrified by the experience, which led her to the realm of yoga. Sarah's yoga journey began with apprehension but quickly transformed into a life-changing event. She learned to control her tension through focused practice, found peace in meditation, and loved the physical asanas that energized her heart.

Sarah's palpitations subsided, her blood pressure returned to normal, and she discovered a new sense of inner serenity. Her experience exemplifies the transforming power of yoga—a holistic approach that not only healed her heart but also revived her whole health.

Finally, the comprehensive approach of yoga to cardiovascular health is a remarkable journey that blends ancient knowledge with current technology. Yoga's diverse advantages range from stress reduction and physical asanas to breath control and mental well-being, making it a strong ally in the search of a healthy heart. Sarah's tale is a strong reminder that yoga practice has the ability to create a heart that beats with vibrancy, resilience, and long-term well-being.

Chapter 2: Foundations of Yoga Practice

In the study of yoga, this chapter serves as the foundation around which the whole practice is built. It goes into the underlying ideas, postures, and breath control methods that support yoga. Practitioners get the information and abilities needed to engage on their transformational yoga journey by thoroughly investigating these fundamental factors. This chapter provides students with the necessary skills to create a comprehensive and heart-centered yoga practice, ranging from mindfulness and alignment through pranayama and asanas.

Mindfulness: The journey starts with mindfulness, which is the discipline of being completely present in the present moment. The profound skill of attentive awareness is presented to readers, developing a deep connection between mind and body. This fundamental component is critical because it not only improves the quality of the practice but also extends its effects beyond the mat and into daily life.

Alignment: The foundation of yoga practice is proper alignment. This chapter addresses the importance of alignment in asanas in great detail. It equips practitioners with the knowledge to grasp the geometry of each pose, assuring safety and efficacy. Aligning the body is about generating room for breath, energy flow, and inner awareness as well as physical form.

Pranayama: The breath, the essential life energy, is reverently studied. Pranayama methods, such as Ujjayi breath and Nadi Shodhana, are introduced. These activities promote regulated and focused breathing, as well as connecting people with their inner rhythms and encouraging emotional equilibrium.

Asanas: Physical postures are the physical manifestation of yoga. This chapter delves into the fundamental asanas, from the Mountain Pose to the Child's Pose. It explains the benefits and drawbacks of each stance, allowing practitioners to select postures that are appropriate for their objectives and physical ability.

Holistic Wellness: Beyond the physical elements, yoga is presented as an approach to holistic wellness. It stresses that yoga goes well beyond the mat, encouraging people toward a healthy lifestyle, conscientious decisions, and emotional well-being.

Heart-Centered Practice: The notion of heart-centered practice is central to this chapter. It encourages people to move and breathe intentionally, compassionately, and lovingly. A heart-centered practice promotes self-acceptance while also encouraging physical and emotional progress.

In essence, Chapter 2 of my book serves as the entry point to a deep journey of self-discovery and well-being via yoga. It gives people the skills they need to embrace yoga holistically, ensuring that it becomes more than simply a fitness regimen but a transforming and heart-centered way of life. The teachings in this chapter will strike a deep chord with readers, laying the groundwork for a joyful and meaningful yoga practice.

Yoga Philosophy and Principles

In Practice Yoga Philosophy: A Way of Life

Yoga philosophy extends beyond the yoga mat and into everyday life. It promotes mindfulness, self-study, and the search of inner joy and tranquility in the face of adversity. Yoga philosophy is a light of hope, guiding us through the complexity of life with grace and tranquility.

Yoga Philosophy and Principles is a philosophical compass that leads readers through the profound and ancient knowledge that supports yoga practice. The rich tapestry of yoga's philosophy and eternal principles are exposed in this chapter, providing a greater knowledge of yoga as more than just a physical practice, but as a comprehensive route to well-being and spiritual enlightenment.

Yoga may be traced back over 5,000 years to the ancient Indus Valley culture in modern-day India. Yoga evolved across time, including the Vedic period, when it was entwined with early religious and spiritual rituals, and the classical period, when Patanjali's Yoga Sutras established many of yoga's philosophical ideas and practices.

Yoga evolved over the years, with new schools and traditions arising. When yoga gurus began to share their teachings with the West in the late nineteenth and early twentieth century, it earned global prominence. Yoga is now practiced all over the world in a variety of forms and ways, all anchored in the deep philosophy and principles that have transcended time and culture.

Yoga is more than simply a physical exercise; it is a deep concept that has guided people for thousands of years on a path of self-discovery, inner tranquility, and spiritual enlightenment. The notion of unity, frequently expressed by the Sanskrit term "yuj," which means to yoke or unite, is at the center of yoga philosophy. This union is multidimensional in that it seeks to unite the individual self (atman) with global awareness (Brahman), and it extends to the interconnection of all beings and the world itself.

Yoga Philosophy's Eightfold Path (Ashtanga)

The eightfold path, often known as Ashtanga, is central to yoga philosophy. This path provides a complete roadmap to having a meaningful and purposeful life. It is made up of eight interrelated limbs, each of which contributes to the individual's holistic development:

1. Yamas (Ethical Principles): These principles, which include non-violence (Ahimsa), honesty (Satya), non-stealing (Asteya), non-excess (Brahmacharya), and non-possessiveness (Aparigraha), regulate ethical behavior.

2. Niyamas (Personal Observances): These comprise purity (Saucha), contentment (Santosha), self-discipline (Tapas), self-study (Svadhyaya), and resignation to a higher power (Ishvara Pranidhana).

3. Asanas (Physical Postures): Physical posture practice not only improves physical flexibility and strength, but it also promotes mental and emotional harmony.

4. Pranayama (Breath Control): Pranayama techniques entail controlling the breath consciously. They aid in the regulation of the vital life energy and the promotion of emotional balance.

5. Pratyahara (Senses Withdrawal): Pratyahara is the practice of turning inward and withdrawing attention from outward stimuli in order to build inner awareness.

6. Dharana (Attention): This limb focuses on developing one-pointed attention in order to prepare the mind for meditation.

7. Dhyana (Meditation): Meditation is a deep state of concentration and awareness in which the mind feels great calm and inner tranquility.

8. Samadhi (Union): Samadhi is the ultimate objective of yoga philosophy, reflecting a profound oneness with the cosmos as well as the realization of one's true nature.

Advaita and Oneness in Yoga Philosophy

The notion of Advaita, which posits the basic oneness of all things, is explored in yoga philosophy. It teaches that apparent barriers between the self and the outside world are really illusions. This deep realization has far-reaching ramifications for human development, empathy, and the cultivation of inner calm.

Karma and Dharma: The Cause-and-Effect Law

The notion of karma, or the law of cause and consequence, is central to yoga philosophy. It teaches that our acts, intentions, and choices determine our fate. It is emphasized that living in accordance with one's dharma, or genuine purpose, leads to meaning, fulfillment, and spiritual advancement.

25 Essential Yoga Poses and Asanas

Yoga positions, also known as asanas, are physical postures that are an important part of the yoga practice. They go beyond simple physical exercise to promote overall well-being by developing flexibility, strength, balance, and mental clarity. Understanding five key yoga positions may be transformational whether you are a novice or a seasoned yogi. We'll look at several major asanas and offer tips on how to do them.

1. *Tadasana* (Mountain Pose)

Benefits: Improves posture, balance, and mental concentration.

How to Get It Done: Keep your feet together, your back straight, and your shoulders relaxed. Engage your core and distribute your weight evenly. Take a deep breath and center yourself.

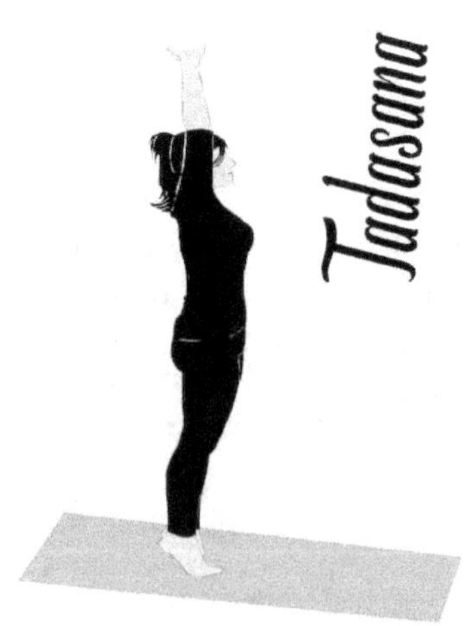

2. Adho Mukha Svanasana (Downward-Facing Dog)

Benefits: Stretches the entire body, strengthens the arms and legs, and helps to relax the mind.

How to Get It Done: Begin on your hands and knees, then elevate your hips toward the ceiling with your palms pressed into the ground. Maintain a hip-width distance between your feet, with your heels lightly pushing on the floor.

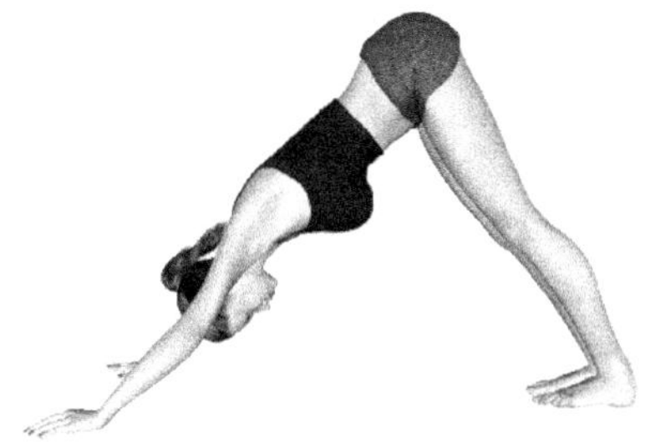

3. Balasana (Child's Pose)

Benefits: Relieves tension by relaxing the back, hips, and shoulders.

How to Get It Done: Sit back on your heels and kneel on the floor, big toes touching. Extend your arms forward, palms down, put your forehead on the mat.

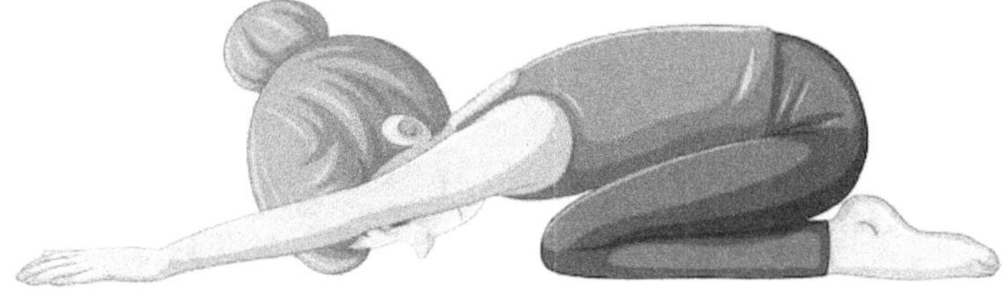

Warrior 1 (Virabhadrasana 1)

Benefits: Increases leg strength and enhances attention.

How to Get It Done: Step forward with one foot and bend the knee at a 90-degree angle. The back foot should be bent at 45 degrees. Raise your arms in front of you, palms facing each other.

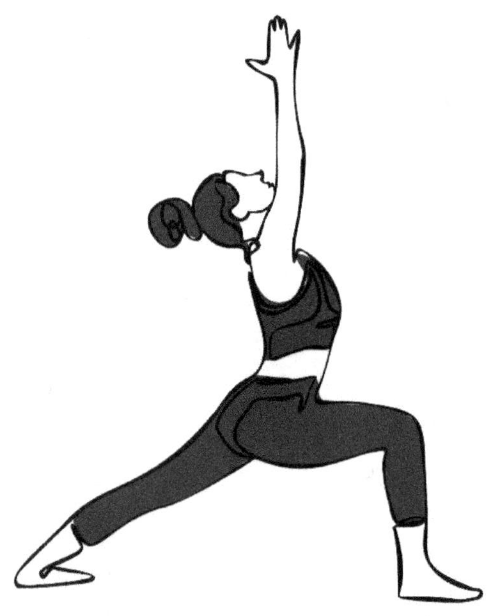

5. Warrior II (Virabhadrasana II)

Benefits: Legs are strengthened and hips are opened.

How to Get It Done: Begin in a wide-legged posture with your arms parallel to the ground. Bend one knee and extend one foot 90 degrees. Examine the front hand.

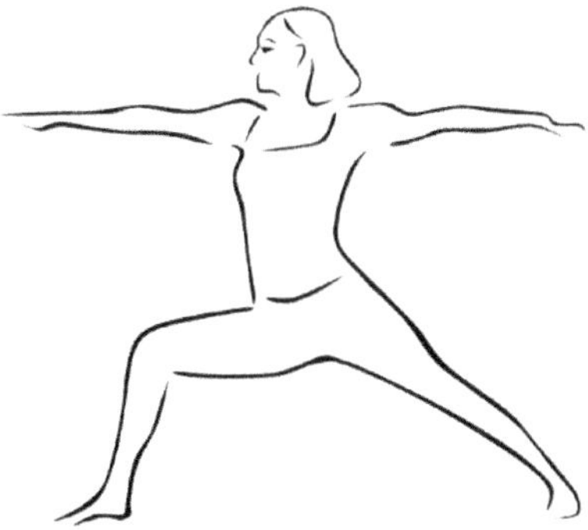

6. Vrikshasana (Tree Pose)

Benefits: include improved balance, focus, and leg strength.

How to Get It Done: Start in Mountain Pose. Place the sole of one foot against the inner thigh of the other leg. In a prayer position, bring your hands to your heart center.

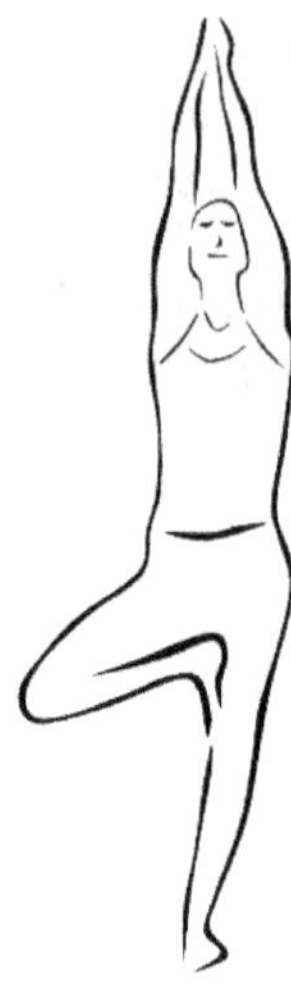

7. Bhujangasana (Cobra Pose)

Benefits: Increases back muscular strength and flexibility.

How to Get It Done: Lie face down with your palms towards your chest. Lift your head and torso off the mat, inhaling as you do so. Look ahead with your elbows slightly bent.

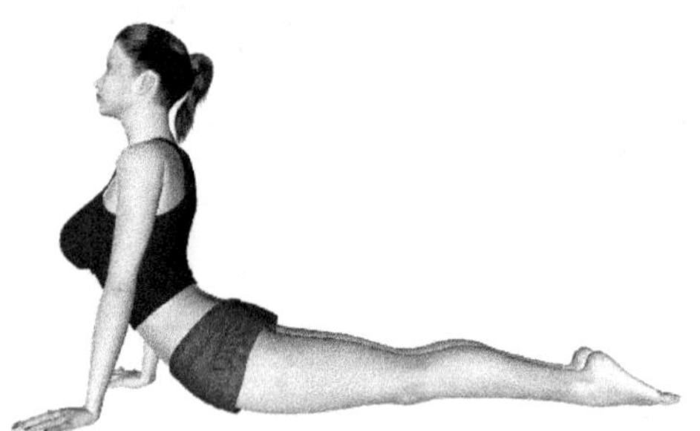

8. Marjaryasana-Bitilasana (Cat-Cow Pose)

Benefits: Increases spinal flexibility and relieves stress.

How to Get It Done: Begin by getting down on your hands and knees. Inhale deeply while arching your back and gazing up (Cow Pose). Exhale while rounding your back and tucking your chin into the Cat Pose.

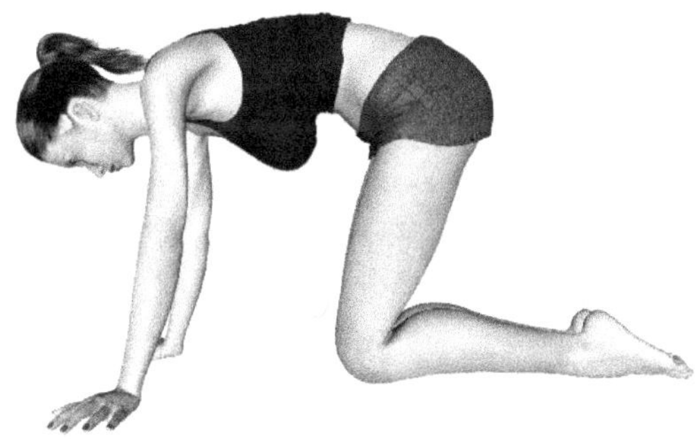

9. Setu Bandha Sarvangasana (Bridge Pose)

Benefits: Increases back, glute, and thigh strength while expanding the chest and improving posture.

How to Get It Done: Lie down on your back with your knees bent and your feet hip-width apart. Lift your hips toward the sky while maintaining your feet and shoulders firmly planted on the ground.

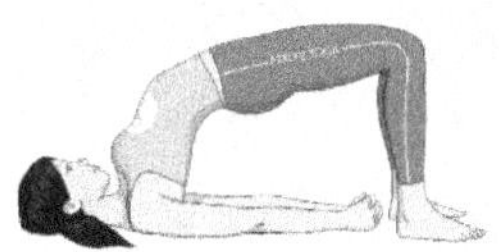

10 Savasana (Corpse Pose]

Benefits: Promotes relaxation and stress reduction.

How to Get It Done: Lie down on your back, arms and legs relaxed. Close your eyes and concentrate on your breathing. Allow your entire body to relax.

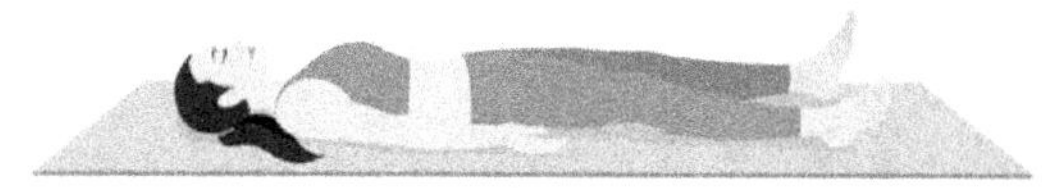

11. Trikonasana (Triangle Pose)

Benefits: Increases leg strength, extends the sides of the body, and improves balance.

How to Get It Done: Place your feet wide apart. Extend one arm all the way down to your ankle or shin, while extending the other arm up toward the sky. Look up or forward.

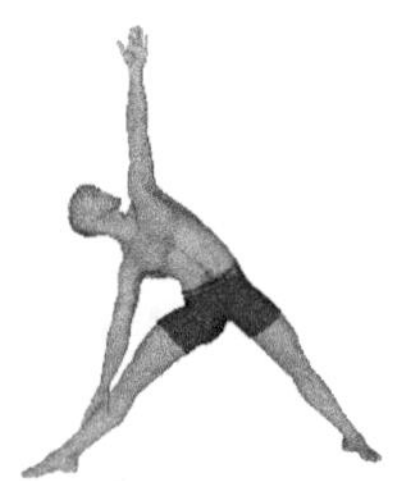

12. Phalakasana (Plank Pose)

Benefits: Tone and strengthens the core, arms and shoulders, and improves posture.

How to Get It Done: Begin in a push-up stance with your arms straight and your shoulders above your wrists. Maintain a straight line from head to heels.

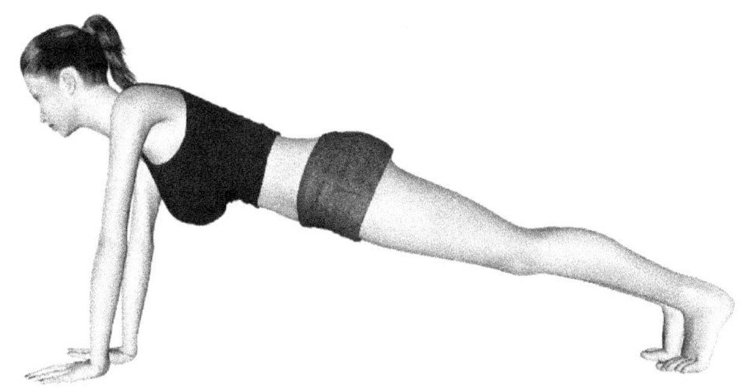

13. Urdhva Mukha Svanasana (Upward-Facing Dog)

Benefits: Arms, chest, and back are strengthened, and the chest is opened.

How to Get It Done: Lie face down with your palms towards your chest. Straighten your arms and elevate your chest off the mat as you exhale. Maintain your feet and hips on the ground.

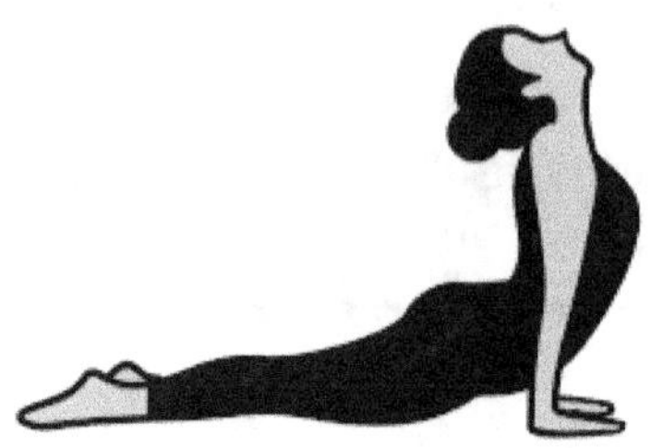

14. Extended Puppy Pose (Uttana Shishosana)

Benefits: This stretch stretches the spine, shoulders, and arms.

How to Get It Done: Begin at the Tabletop position. Walking your hands forward, drop your torso and forehead to the mat, and keep your hips above your knees.

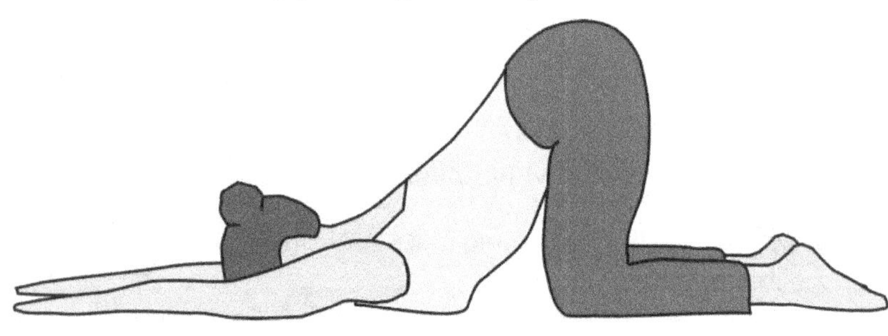

15. Navasana (Boat Pose)

Benefits: Improves core and hip flexor strength.

How to Get It Done: Sit with your knees bent and your feet flat on the floor. Balance on your sitting bones by leaning back slightly and lifting your feet off the ground. Extend your arms forward or keep them close to your hips.

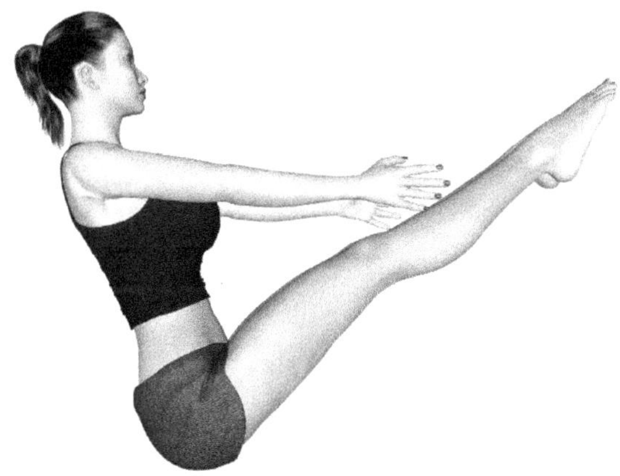

16. Ustrasana (Camel Pose)

Benefits include stretching the front of the body, improving posture, and opening the chest.

How to Get It Done: Kneel, keeping your knees hip-width apart. Reach back and place your hands on your heels, arching your back and raising your chest.

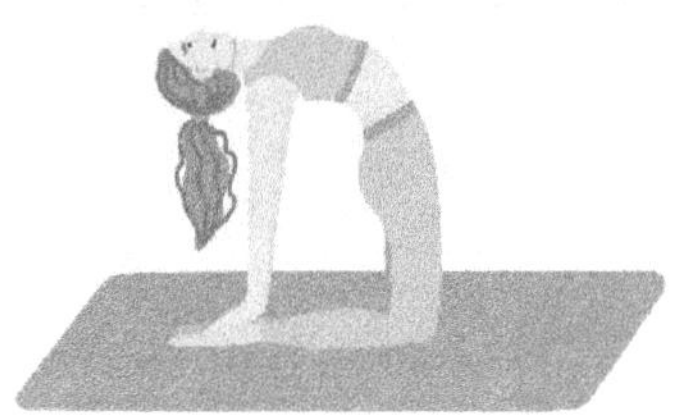

17. Malasana (Garland Pose)

Benefits: Strengthens and tones the ankles and lower back.

How to Get It Done: Squat with your feet wider than hip-width apart and your toes turned out slightly. Bring your palms together at your heart and gently push your knees apart with your elbows.

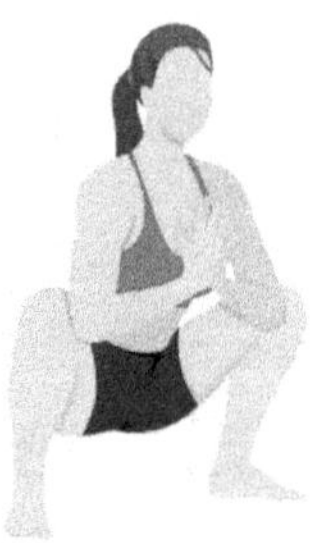

18. Matsyasana (Fish Pose)

Benefits: Stretches the front of the neck, opens the chest and throat, and improves posture.

How to Get It Done: Lie down on your back with your legs outstretched. Place your hands, palms down, beneath your hips. Lift your chest and arch your back, softly resting your head on the ground.

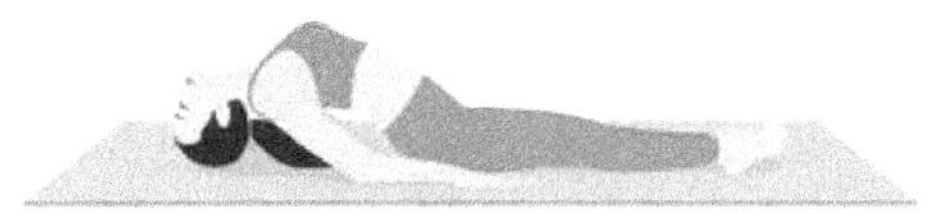

19. Ananda Balasana (Happy Baby Pose)

Benefits: Stretches the hamstrings and relaxes the hips and lower back.

How to Get It Done: Lie back, bend your knees toward your armpits, and hold the outsides of your feet. Pull your knees gently toward the floor beside your torso.

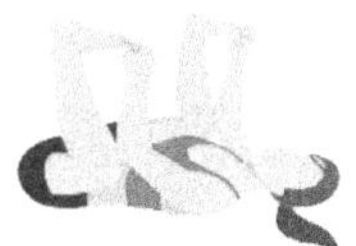

20. Eka Pada Rajakapotasana (Pigeon Pose)

Benefits: Deeply stretches the hips and thighs.

How to Get It Done: Begin in the Downward-Facing Dog position. Bring one knee up to your chest and position it behind your wrist, inclined outward. Slide your other leg back and stretch it behind you. Fold forward and square your hips.

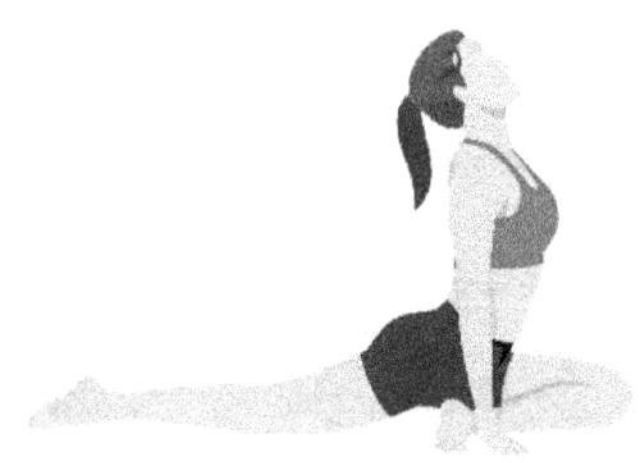

21. Sarvangasana (Shoulder Stand)

Benefits: Increases circulation, reduces tension, and strengthens shoulders and neck.

How to Get It Done: Lie on your back and raise your legs and hips, using your hands to support your lower back. Straighten your legs and extend them toward the ceiling.

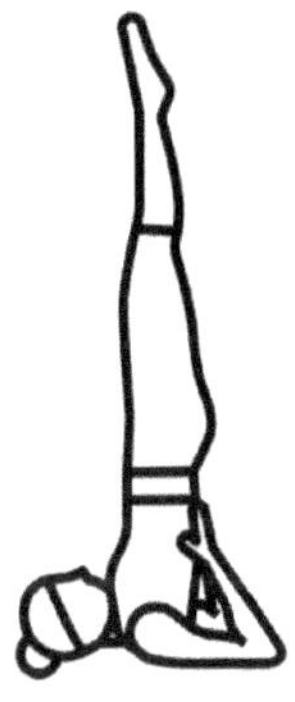

22. Bakasana (Crow Pose)

Benefits: Arms and wrists are strengthened, balance is improved, and core strength is built.

How to Get It Done: Begin in a squat, place your hands on the floor, and lean forward, moving your weight onto your hands and elevating your feet off the ground.

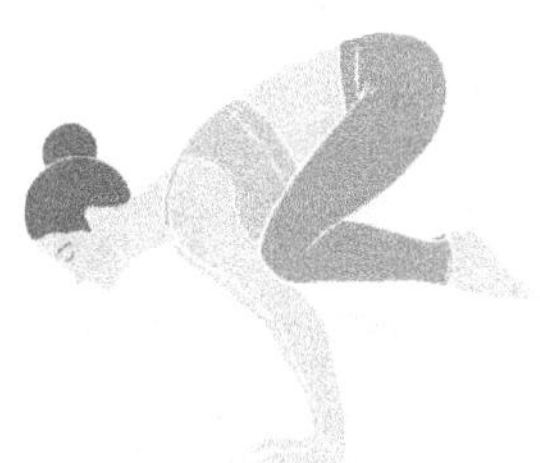

23. Paschimottanasana (Seated Forward Bend)

Benefits: Stretches and soothes the whole rear of the body.

How to Get It Done: Sit with legs extended. To reach your toes, hinge at your hips. Maintain a long spine and a chest that reaches all the way to your toes.

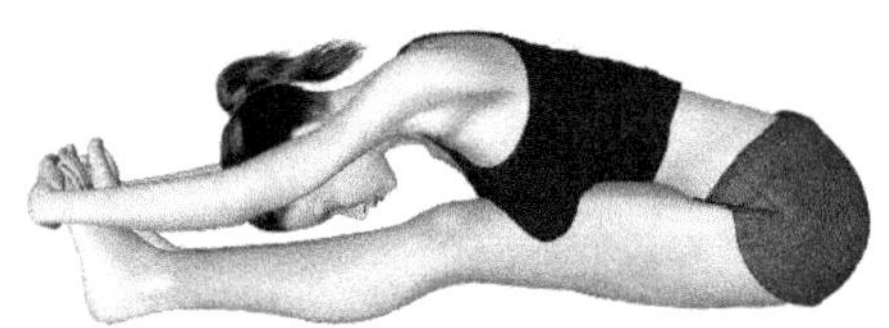

24. Uttanasana (Standing Forward Bend)

Benefits: Stretches the hamstrings and spine, lowers tension, and relaxes the mind.

How to Get It Done: Place your feet hip-width apart. Fold forward, hinge at the hips, and reach for your toes or the floor. If necessary, keep your knees slightly bent.

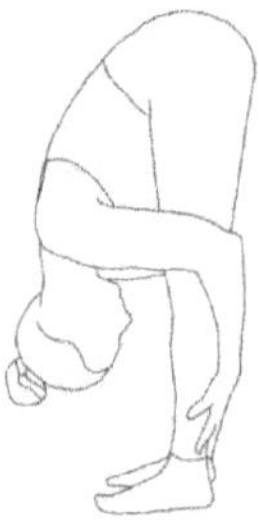

25. Sphinx Pose (Salamba Bhujangasana)

Benefits: Strengthens the spine and opens up the chest.

How to Get It Done: Lie down on your stomach, forearms on the ground, elbows under your shoulders. Engage your back muscles and lift your chest.

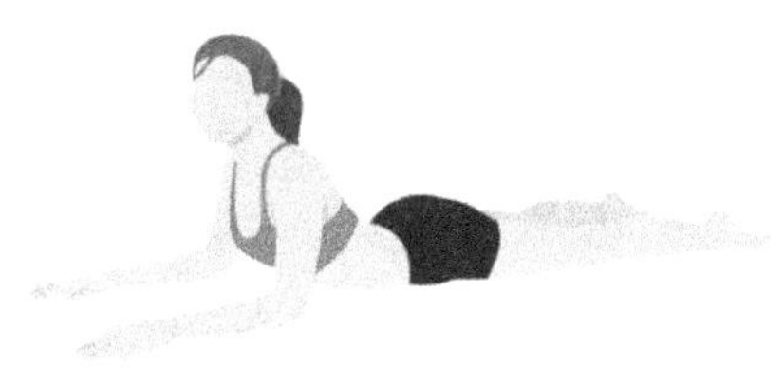

Achieving Yoga Poses: Success Strategies

Practice on a regular basis: Consistency is essential. Make time to practice these postures on a regular basis to increase your flexibility and strength.

Pay Attention to Your Body: Take note of your body's cues. Instead, then forcing a position, relax into it gently.

Use Props: Props like as blocks, straps, and bolsters can help you achieve perfect alignment and support in your postures.

Mindfully Breathe: Breathing is an essential aspect of yoga. Throughout each stance, take slow, deep breaths.

Seek direction: For individualized direction and adjustments, consider attending yoga classes, viewing instructional videos, or seeing a professional yoga instructor.

Modify as Needed: Always feel free to modify poses if you have physical limitations or injuries. Yoga may be adjusted to meet the needs of each individual.

Incorporating these important yoga positions into your practice may improve both your physical and emotional health. Always keep in mind that yoga is a journey, not a destination. You may uncover the transforming power of these core asanas with patience, attention, and devotion, promoting comprehensive health and inner peace.

Pranayama and Breathwork for Heart Health: A Path to Vitality

The ancient practice of yoga offers a calming salve for the spirit in the hectic tapestry of modern life, where stress often weaves its threads into our everyday experiences. It's a route back to tranquility, harmony, and a deep connection to our inner selves.

The technique of breathwork, or Pranayama, is one of the most transforming components of yoga, particularly in terms of heart health.

Consider this: A lady called Sarah found herself enmeshed in the unrelenting demands of her career, family, and daily commutes in the vivid turmoil of a thriving metropolis. Her heart carried the weight of her life's responsibilities, both literally and symbolically. Stress was a regular companion, and her blood pressure began to rise, indicating impending disaster.

Sarah found the astonishing influence of Pranayama on heart health at this critical point. Her story teaches us about the healing power of mindful breathing and its enormous influence on our cardiovascular health.

Understanding Pranayama: The Life Breath

Pranayama is an ancient yogic technique that focuses on breath control and regulation. It is based on the idea that the breath is more than just a biological function, but rather a link between the physical body and the subtle forces that regulate our vitality.

Pranayama refers to a range of breathing methods, each having its own set of advantages for heart health:

1. Deep Diaphragmatic Breathing: Sarah's journey began with deep diaphragmatic breathing. In this simple yet effective method, inhale deeply through the nose, expand the diaphragm, and exhale gently through pursed lips. It quickly promotes a relaxing reaction, decreasing blood pressure and tension.

2. Ujjayi Breathing: Sarah eventually included Ujjayi breathing, sometimes known as "ocean breath" because of its peaceful, rhythmic sound. This approach not only relaxes the mind but also improves cardiac function and circulation.

3. Anulom Vilom (Alternate Nostril Breathing): Sarah adopted Anulom Vilom, a Pranayama method that balances the body's energy, as she progressed in her practice. It improves heart health by lowering cardiac strain and increasing blood flow.

4. Bhastrika (Bellows Breath): Sarah used Bhastrika, a powerful breathing method, to revitalize her heart and rejuvenate her body. This vigorous activity improves cardiovascular endurance and promotes heart health by increasing circulation.

5. Kapalabhati (Skull Shining Breath): A cleaning breath, Kapalabhati became a part of Sarah's daily practice. This therapy removes toxins from the body, which can lead to heart disease if not addressed.

Sarah's Success Story: A Changed Heart

Sarah's Pranayama journey was nothing short of remarkable. As she committed to regular breathwork and Pranayama, amazing changes began to take place. Her stress levels dropped, and she discovered a new feeling of inner serenity and resilience.

The effect on her heart health was equally impressive. Her blood pressure, which had previously been a source of worry, had now settled within a healthy range.

The secret was in her conscious control of her breath, which created a relaxation response, lowering the release of stress hormones and relieving the strain on her heart.

Sarah's achievement is not unusual. Scientific studies have continuously shown a strong link between Pranayama and heart health. Controlled breathing has been demonstrated to:

- Lower Blood Pressure: Pranayama, like it did for Sarah, can result in considerable blood pressure reductions, making it an excellent supplemental therapy for hypertension management.

- Reduce Stress: Chronic stress has been linked to heart disease. Pranayama is a natural stress reliever that calms the mind and lowers the wear and strain on the heart.

- Improve Oxygenation: Pranayama methods improve circulation and oxygen flow to key organs, including the heart.

- Improve Heart Rate Variability (HRV): A healthy HRV is associated with improved heart health. Pranayama has a favorable effect on HRV, boosting cardiovascular resiliency.

The Effectiveness of Consistency and Mindfulness

Sarah's metamorphosis was the product of regular effort and focused breathing, rather than an instant miracle. This is an important lesson for everyone interested in improving their heart health via Pranayama.

Pranayama might be a game changer for your heart if you include it into your everyday practice. Even a few minutes of intentional breathing each day might have a significant impact. Whether you're new to yoga or an experienced practitioner, the path to heart health starts with your next breath.

Remember that the power is within you as you begin on your own road to heart health with Pranayama. Pause for a moment, breathe mindfully, and nourish your heart with each inhale and exhale.

Let Sarah's tale serve as a light of hope and encouragement to others. Allow it to serve as a reminder that the ancient knowledge of yoga, distilled in the discipline of breathwork, has the power to alter not just your heart, but your whole existence. The breath is your most powerful ally on the road to vitality and well-being.

With each breath, you get closer to a healthier heart, a more peaceful mind, and a more vibrant existence. The trip begins with the next inhale—enjoy it, appreciate it, and allow it to guide you to the heart-healthy lifestyle you deserve.

Chapter 3: Yoga as a Stress-Reduction Technique

Stress and Its Effect on the Heart: Unraveling the Link

Stress has become an ever-present companion for many people in the maelstrom of modern life. It's the uninvited guest at the table, the shadow that follows us around all day. While stress is a natural reaction to life's difficulties, its prolonged presence can have a negative impact on our heart health.

Let's go on a trip to untangle the complex link between stress and the heart, demystifying its influence in a way that everyone can understand.

Nature's Alarm System: The Stress Response

To understand how stress affects the heart, we must first know the body's extraordinary stress response. When confronted with a perceived threat, whether it's a pressing work deadline or an unexpected shock, our bodies go into "fight or flight" mode.

This instinctual response fills our system with stress chemicals, principally cortisol and adrenaline. These hormones prepare us to confront or flee the imagined danger. Our heart rate accelerates, our blood pressure rises, and our energy reserves are depleted.

The Silent Saboteur: Chronic Stress

While the stress reaction is necessary for survival, it has evolved into a persistent, chronic force in modern life. Our stress response is kept on high alert by the daily grind, financial difficulties, and societal demands. Chronic stress has a significant influence on our heart health.

1. High Blood Pressure: Chronic stress contributes to high blood pressure. High blood pressure (hypertension) stresses the heart over time, increasing the risk of heart disease and stroke.

2. Raise in Inflammation: Stress causes inflammation in the body. Persistent artery inflammation can lead to the development of atherosclerosis, or the formation of plaque in the arteries, compromising heart health even further.

3. Heart Rhythm Disturbances: Stress can cause arrhythmias by disrupting the heart's rhythm. Severe arrhythmias are potentially fatal.

4. Coronary Artery Spasms: Stress can cause spasms in the coronary arteries, which feed blood to the heart muscle. These spasms can restrict blood supply to the heart, resulting in chest discomfort or angina.

5. Unhealthy Coping techniques: When faced with chronic stress, many people resort to unhealthy coping techniques such as overeating, excessive alcohol use, or smoking, all of which are harmful to their heart health.

Mind and Heart: A Potent Combination

The relationship between the mind and the heart is fundamental. When stress persists, it can have an impact on not just the physical but also the emotional and mental elements of heart health.

1. Psychological Stress: The emotional toll of chronic stress can lead to disorders such as depression and anxiety, which are risk factors for heart disease in and of themselves.

2. Behavioral Impact: When people are stressed, they frequently engage in heart-harming behaviors such as poor food choices, lack of exercise, and drug misuse.

Breaking the Chain: Stress Management for Heart Health

The first step toward breaking the chain is to understand the relationship between stress and heart health. Here are some simple strategies to deal with stress and preserve your heart:

1. Deep Breathing: Breathe deeply and diaphragmatically to stimulate your body's relaxation response.

2. Exercise on a Regular Basis: Physical exercise produces endorphins, which assist to alleviate stress. Most days, aim for at least 30 minutes of moderate activity.

3. Mindfulness and Meditation: These practices can assist you in remaining grounded, reducing stress, and improving your mental well-being.

4. Healthy Diet: A well-balanced diet rich in fruits, vegetables, whole grains, and lean meats promotes both physical and emotional well-being.

5. Adequate Sleep: Make quality sleep a priority to help your body recover from stress.

6. Seek Help: When stress becomes unbearable, don't be afraid to call out to friends, family, or a mental health professional.

Finally, a Message from the Heart

Stress is an unavoidable aspect of life, but it does not have to be a constant load on our hearts. We can safeguard our most critical organ by understanding the delicate dance between stress and heart health.

Remember that your heart is not simply a physical force, but it is also the seat of your emotions and well-being. Allow this information to function as a compass, directing you toward a heart-healthy, stress-resilient route as you face life's obstacles. Accept leisure, seek balance, and treasure your heart—it's the beat of your existence.

Yoga for Stress Reduction

Stress has become an unpleasant companion for many in our fast-paced and often chaotic environment. It infiltrates our lives, negatively impacting our physical health, emotional well-being, and general quality of life. This investigation delves into the profound practice of yoga as a potent stress-reduction tool, backed by the inspiring narrative of Sarah, a patient whose life was altered by yoga.

Understanding Stress: A Modern Epidemic

Stress is a ubiquitous human experience that serves as an adaptive reaction to life's difficulties. Chronic stress, on the other hand, has become an epidemic in our modern culture, slowly destroying our health and happiness. Work, family, financial constraints, and an onslaught of information may leave us feeling overwhelmed and imbalanced.

Unmanaged stress has far-reaching consequences:

1. Physical Toll: Physical signs of stress include headaches, muscular tightness, and digestive difficulties. It leads to chronic diseases such as hypertension and heart disease.

2. Mental Strain: Prolonged stress can cause anxiety, sadness, and cognitive problems, affecting our ability to think clearly and make informed judgments.

3. Emotional Upheaval: Stress may exacerbate emotions, making us more prone to rage, irritation, and melancholy. It has the potential to disrupt relationships and degrade our feeling of well-being.

Yoga's Ancient Wisdom

Enter yoga, a practice that provides a refuge of quiet in the midst of contemporary life's maelstrom. Yoga is a comprehensive method that harmonizes the body, mind, and spirit that is based on ancient Indian philosophy. At its heart is the conviction that real well-being is more than only the absence of sickness, but also a condition of vital health and inner harmony.

A Journey to Inner Peace: Sarah's Transformation

Sarah's experience demonstrates the therapeutic effect of yoga for stress reduction. She sought peace in the practice of yoga from me, her physician; she was suffering from chronic stress. Her journey began on a yoga mat, but it quickly expanded beyond the physical.

1. Physical Liberation: Sarah's body began to release deeply held tension via the gentle flow of yoga postures (asanas). Her muscles eased and she felt more at ease.

2. Breath as a Bridge: Sarah was exposed to the profound skill of mindful breathing (Pranayama) through yoga. This practice became her safety net. Deep, deliberate breaths carried her from the confusion of her mind to the peace inside.

3. Mindful Awareness: Sarah learned to examine her thoughts without judgment via the practice of mindfulness, a basic concept of yoga. This newly discovered self-awareness enabled her to break free from the cycle of worry and anxiety.

4. Emotional Resilience: As Sarah's yoga experience progressed, she found that her emotional reactions to challenges were more measured. Yoga provided her with the tools she needed to face problems with grace and composure.

5. Community and Support: Sarah found consolation in the welcoming community of other yogis. She realized she wasn't alone in her quest for stress relief and mental well-being.

The Science of Yoga's Stress-Reducing Properties

Yoga's anti-stress benefits are not only anecdotal. Scientific studies have confirmed the multiple advantages of this old practice:

1. Cortisol Regulation: Yoga has been demonstrated to lower cortisol, the body's major stress hormone, resulting in feelings of calm and relaxation.

2. Neurological Changes: According to neuroimaging research, regular yoga practice can affect brain areas related with stress and emotion management.

3. Increased Resilience: Yoga promotes emotional resilience, helping people to recover more quickly from challenges.

4. Improved Heart Health: Yoga supports cardiovascular health by decreasing blood pressure and heart rate, especially in the face of stress.

A Call to Action: Discovering Your Inner Oasis

Yoga is a stress-reduction method that is open to everyone, regardless of age, fitness ability, or expertise. It is a voyage that allows you to explore the landscape of your own body and mind, cultivating an inner feeling of harmony.

Remember Sarah's story while you explore the world of yoga. Allow it to serve as an example of the transformational potential of this ancient practice. Whether you lay out your mat at home or attend a yoga class, you are taking a step toward increased well-being and inner serenity.

May you discover a sanctuary in the calming embrace of yoga, where tension melts, leaving behind a profound feeling of tranquility and a heart that beats to the rhythm of serenity.

Yoga Nidra with Guidance for Deep Relaxation

Moments of pure relaxation might feel like rare diamonds in the middle of our fast-paced, demanding existence. Yoga Nidra, an ancient technique that guides us to a state of profound relaxation and inner silence, provides a road to these times. In this inquiry, we'll learn about the essence of Yoga Nidra, its numerous advantages, and how to harness its power for deep relaxation.

Understanding Yoga Nidra: Sleep Yoga

Yoga Nidra, often known as "yogic sleep," is a method of guided meditation. Despite its name, it is a technique of profound relaxation and heightened awareness rather than rest. It has grown from old yogic traditions into a disciplined practice for current times.

Yoga Nidra's core rests in its capacity to take practitioners to the point between consciousness and sleep, when deep relaxation occurs. The body and mind feel a tremendous relief of stress in this condition, and the subconscious mind becomes open to good impulses.

Yoga Nidra Stages: A Guided Journey

Yoga Nidra is often divided into phases, each of which is intended to create a distinct level of relaxation and awareness. While techniques may differ, the fundamental framework stays the same:

1. *Setting an Intention*: The practice begins with the establishment of a sankalpa, or deep intention or commitment. Throughout the practice, this leads the subconscious mind.

2. *Body Scan*: You'll be taken through a methodical scan of your body, paying attention to each component and releasing tension mindfully.

3. *Breath Awareness*: Next, you'll concentrate on your breathing, becoming aware of its natural rhythm.

4. *Emotional Awareness*: The practice frequently entails investigating and accepting your feelings in order to promote emotional healing and balance.

5. *Visualization*: Guided imagery may be utilized to excite your senses and move your mind to a relaxing environment.

6. *Sankalpa Reinforcement:* Your initial purpose is revisited, strengthening it in your subconscious's fertile ground.

7. *Rotation of Consciousness*: This step includes mentally "visiting" various sections of your body, which promotes relaxation and heightened awareness.

8. *Return to Wakefulness:* The exercise culminates with a gentle return to full wakefulness, sometimes with a sensation of renewal and tranquility.

Yoga Nidra's Healing Potential

Yoga Nidra has several and significant advantages for your physical, mental, and emotional well-being:

1. *Stress Reduction*: Yoga Nidra is an effective stress reliever. It stimulates the relaxation response, which reduces the synthesis of stress hormones such as cortisol.

2. *Better Sleep*: Regular practice can relieve insomnia and improve peaceful sleep, making it an invaluable aid for anyone suffering from sleep problems.

3. *Increased Focus and Creativity*: By reducing the mind's continuous chatter, Yoga Nidra improves mental clarity and creativity.

4. *Emotional Healing*: It offers a secure environment for exploring and resolving emotional concerns, resulting in increased emotional resilience.

5. *Pain Management:* Yoga Nidra can help with chronic pain by relaxing you and changing your perception of pain.

6. *Mind-Body link*: The exercise increases your awareness of the mind-body link, allowing you to recover holistically.

A Guided Practice for Harnessing the Power of Yoga Nidra

To get the most out of Yoga Nidra, it's best to practice with a guided audio recording or a certified instructor. You may try this reduced version:

1. Find a quiet, comfortable place to lie down on your back, arms slightly apart and palms facing up.

2. Close your eyes and breathe deeply and calmly.

3. Make a goal for your practice. What do you want to grow or release? Make a concise, positive remark in the present tense.

4. Begin mentally scanning your body, beginning at your toes and working your way up. As you move, consciously release tension from each region of your body.

5. Pay attention to your breathing. Observe its natural rhythm without attempting to manipulate it.

6. Allow any ideas or feelings to arise and pass without judgement. Return your attention to your breathing.

7. If you have an intention, say it three times silently to yourself.

8. Return your awareness to your surroundings gradually, wriggling your fingers and toes, and then softly open your eyes.

Yoga Nidra is an invitation to go inside, to a place of deep relaxation and self-discovery. It's a haven of calm in the middle of life's turmoil—a place to find comfort, renewal, and clarity.

Remember that Yoga Nidra is more than just a relaxing method; it is also a portal to self-transformation. It may become a steady partner on your quest to inner serenity and well-being with frequent practice.

Chapter 4: Yoga Sequences for Heart Health

The heart is a critical pillar of vitality in the search for complete well-being. Yoga sequences designed for heart health provide a comprehensive approach to caring for this crucial organ. These sequences integrate old yoga knowledge with current cardiovascular wellness principles to provide a balanced practice for heart-centered health.

Yoga's effectiveness in boosting heart health stems from its capacity to unite the mind and body. Yoga practices promote a mind-body connection, which helps control blood pressure, decrease inflammation, and improve overall cardiovascular function.

Yoga sequences for heart health are not a one-size-fits-all solution; they may be customized to meet the demands and fitness levels of each individual. All of them share a dedication to supporting the heart, not just as a physical organ, but also as the emotional and spiritual basis of our existence.

You can start on a path toward heart-centered life by incorporating yoga practices into your everyday routine. These sequences offer a path to understanding and caring to the demands of your heart, establishing emotional balance, and promoting physical health. May your heart blossom with vigor, strength, and an abiding feeling of well-being as you accept the wisdom of these sequences.

Energize Your Heart: A Morning Yoga Routine

A new day is a blessing, an opportunity to set the tone for the hours ahead. A morning yoga program designed to awaken your heart and mind might be a powerful way to accept this gift. We will dig into the essence of a heart-energizing morning practice, replete with 10 invigorating yoga postures and instructions on how to incorporate them into your daily ritual, in this inquiry.

A Morning Yoga Routine's Essence

Morning yoga is more than simply physical postures; it is a comprehensive practice that includes movement, breath, and awareness. Its goal is to instill vigor, clarity, and a feeling of purpose into your day. This exercise unifies the body and mind, laying the groundwork for a healthy and heart-centered life.

10 Energizing Morning Yoga Poses

1. Tadasana (Mountain Pose):

-Stand erect with your feet hip-width apart.

- Center your weight on your feet and rise through your crown.

- Take several deep breaths and set an intention for the day.

2. Surya Namaskar (Sun Salutation):

- This flowing routine warms up the entire body.

- Forward folds, lunges, and upward-facing dog positions should all be included.

3. Cat-Cow Stretch:

- Begin on your hands and knees.

- Inhale deeply and arch your back (Cow Pose).

- Exhale and circle your spine (Cat Pose).

- To wake up your spine, repeat this mild flow multiple times.

4. Downward-Facing Dog (Adho Mukha Svanasana):

- Push your hips up and back from a plank posture.

- Form an inverted V with your body.

- Stretch your hamstrings and spine.

5. Child's position (Balasana):

- Relax and stretch your back and shoulders in this position.

- Extend your arms in front of you and sink your hips back into your heels.

6. Virabhadrasana II (Warrior II):

- Step one foot back into a lunge, spreading your arms out to the sides.

- Look at your front hand.

- Contract your leg muscles to build strength and stability.

7. Triangle Pose (Trikonasana):

- Straighten your front leg and reach forward, dropping your hand to your shin or a block from Warrior II.

- Raise your opposing arm toward the heavens.

- This position expands your heart and stretches your sides.

8. Bridge Pose (Setu Bandhasana):

- Lie on your back with your knees bent and your feet hip-width apart.

- Raise your hips to the sky while working your glutes and heart center.

- Use your hands to support your lower back.

9. Ustrasana (Camel Pose):

- Kneel with your knees hip-width apart.

- Retract your steps, resting your hands on your heels or lower back.

- Point your heart toward the heavens.

10. Seated Meditation:

- Finish your routine by sitting for a few minutes.

- Close your eyes, concentrate on your breathing, and establish a good purpose for the day.

Including Yoga in Your Morning Routine

1. Set Your Alarm: Schedule your practice time each morning, and set an alarm if necessary to ensure you have enough time.

2. Prepare Your Space: Clear a peaceful, clutter-free location in which to practice. Set out your yoga mat and any props you'll be using.

3. Begin Slowly: Begin with a shorter routine and gradually increase the number of postures and duration as your practice progresses.

4. Mindful Movement: As you go through each posture, pay attention to your breath and sensations. Allow distractions to disappear and concentrate on the current moment.

5. Consistency Is Key: Creating a consistent morning routine will intensify the advantages over time.

Energizing your heart with a morning yoga session is a daily gift you offer to yourself. It's a self-care practice that nourishes your body, clears your mind, and sets a pleasant tone for the rest of your day. Accept this exercise as a holy rite, and allow it to pour vigor and meaning into your life. Now is the right time to head back to Chapter 2 of this book. Look out for those poses and be consistent with them. You're going to thank me later.

Rejuvenate and Relax: Evening Yoga Practices

As the sun sets and the day comes to an end, it's the ideal moment to enter a quiet and restorative frame of mind. Evening yoga practices are a peaceful way to unwind, release the stresses of the day, and prepare both body and mind for a restful night's sleep. We'll dig into the essence of nighttime yoga practices in this inquiry, replete with fifteen relaxing yoga positions and instructions on how to incorporate them into your bedtime ritual.

The Importance of Evening Yoga Practices

Evening yoga practices work as a transition point between the activity of the day and the tranquility of the night. They are intentional pauses that invite you to let go of the outside world and reconnect with your inner self. Gentle movement, calming breathwork, and deep relaxation are included into these activities to prepare you for a restful night's sleep.

15 Relaxing Yoga Poses for the Evening

1. Child's Pose (Balasana):

   - Begin on your knees, then drop your torso forward with your arms outstretched.

   - Place your forehead on the mat and let your spine to relax.

2. Cat-Cow Stretch:

   - On hands and knees, inhale while arching your back (Cow Pose) and exhale while rounding your back (Cat Pose).

   - Repeat this action to warm up the spine.

3. Uttanasana (Standing Forward Bend):

   - From a standing position, hinge at your hips, allowing your upper body to fold forward.

   - Relax your head and neck, and stretch your spine.

4. Low Lunge (Anjaneyasana):

   - Take a step forward into a lunge stance.

   - Squeeze your hip flexors and feel the slight stretch.

5. Butterfly Pose (Baddha Konasana):

   - Lie on your back with your feet together and your knees apart.

   - Gently push your knees toward the floor while maintaining a straight spine.

6. Supine Twist:

   - Lie on your back with your arms at your sides.

   - Bring one leg up to your chest and cross it across your torso, twisting your spine.

7. Legs Up the Wall (Viparita Karani):

   - Bring your hips up against a wall and extend your legs upward.

   - This position encourages relaxation and might help with leg tiredness.

8. Ananda Balasana (Happy Baby):

   - Lie on your back and pull your knees to your chest.

   - Rock from side to side while holding your feet.

9. Supta Baddha Konasana (Reclining Bound Angle Pose):

   - Lie on your back, bend your knees, and allow the soles of your feet meet.

   - Take your time with this easy hip opener.

10. Paschimottanasana (Seated Forward Bend):

- Sit with your legs outstretched in front of you.

- Keep your spine extended and hinge at your hips to reach towards your toes.

11. Corpse Pose (Savasana):

- Lie on your back with your arms at your sides.

- Concentrate on relaxing every muscle in your body.

12. Nadi Shodhana (Alternate Nostril Breathing):

- Sit comfortably, shut one nostril, and inhale.

- Then exhale from the other nostril.

- This approach relaxes the mind and restores energy balance.

13. Three-Part Breath (Dirga Pranayama):

- Inhale deeply into your lower belly, ribs, and upper chest.

- Exhale in the other direction.

- This breathing technique encourages relaxation and attention.

14. Belly Breathing:

- Lie on your back with one hand on your stomach.

- Take deep breaths into your tummy, feeling it rise and fall with each one.

15. Counted Breathing:

- Inhale for four counts, hold for four counts, exhale for four counts, and hold for four counts.

- This approach aids in the regulation of your breath and the relaxation of your thoughts.

Integrating Yoga into Your Evening Routine

1. Select a Quiet Area: Locate a tranquil place where you will not be disturbed.

2. Make a Gentle Intention: Think about your day and make a gentle intention for a restful night.

3. Dim the Lights: Lowering the lights creates a relaxing ambience.

4. Mindful Movement: Move attentively through each posture, paying attention to your breath.

5. Relaxation and Stillness: Spend a significant amount of time in Savasana, letting your body and mind to unwind.

6. Consistency: For maximum outcomes, establish a consistent nightly routine.

Evening yoga is a self-care gift, a peaceful haven that promotes your well-being and prepares you for healthy sleep. May your evenings become a sanctuary of serenity and renewal as you embrace these relaxing postures and focused breathwork, setting the tone for peaceful nights and revitalized mornings.

Specialized Sequences for Heart Conditions

Individual demands differ greatly when it comes to heart health. Yoga sequences designed specifically for heart issues provide a sophisticated and focused approach to increasing cardiovascular well-being. In this exploration, we'll dig into the substance of these sequences, comprehending their significance and giving 10 unique sequences suited for people with varied heart health concerns. We'll also provide tips on how readers may safely and efficiently implement these sequences into their practice.

Specialized Sequences' Importance

Heart issues can range from hypertension and coronary artery disease to arrhythmias and cardiac failure. Specialized yoga sequences take these variances into account and concentrate on certain areas of heart health, such as:

1. Heart Muscle Strengthening: Some disorders may necessitate increased heart muscle strength and endurance.

2. Improving Circulation: Improving blood flow can be critical for people who have specific cardiac difficulties.

3. Managing Stress: Stress reduction is important for preserving heart health.

4. Mindful Breathwork: Some sequences emphasize pranayama techniques to increase lung capacity and decrease anxiety.

5. Flexibility and Range of Motion: Gentle stretching may help with conditions such as angina or a recent heart attack.

6. Balancing Blood Pressure: Hypertension treatment is an important consideration.

10 Specialized Yoga Sequences for Cardiovascular Health

1. Hypertension Helper:

- Focuses on stress reduction and blood pressure lowering postures.

- Uses breath control methods such as Alternate Nostril Breathing.

2. Heart Strengthening Flow:

- Focuses on postures that gently stretch the heart muscle.

- Backbends such as Cobra Pose are included for heart conditioning.

3. Circulation Booster:

- Improves blood flow via dynamic postures and breathwork.

- Incorporates positions like as Warrior II to promote circulation.

4. Angina Alleviation Sequence:

- Gentle stretches to relieve chest pain.

- Contains the Chest Opener Pose for chest comfort.

5. Arrhythmia Awareness:

- Mindful breathing techniques to relieve anxiety and regulate heart rhythm.

- Emphasizes relaxing positions such as Child's Pose.

6. Heart Attack Recovery Routine:

- Progressive postures to regain strength following a heart attack.

- Chair Pose is used for progressive muscular development.

7. Management of Heart Failure:

- Low-intensity sequences to minimize overexertion.

- Includes sitting positions such as sitting Forward Bend.

8. Coronary Artery Care:

- Pose and stretch to preserve flexibility and prevent plaque development.

- Triangle Pose is included for side body stretching.

9. Stress Buster Sequence:

- Techniques for stress reduction through restorative postures.

- For relaxation, do positions like Legs Up the Wall.

10. Holistic Heart Health:

- A multifaceted approach to heart health.

- This practice incorporates mild positions, attentive breathwork, and meditation.

Adding Specialized Sequences to Your Practice

1. Consult a Professional: Prior to starting any specialized sequence, consult a medical professional to ensure it's safe and suitable for your condition.

2. Mindful Practice: During sequences, pay special attention to your body. If you feel any discomfort or pain, stop immediately.

3. Consistency: To reap the advantages, practice on a regular yet gentle basis. Always emphasize safety above overexertion.

4. Listen to Your Body: Your needs may change over time. Adapt your practice as needed.

5. Professional Guidance: If feasible, practice with a competent yoga instructor who is versed in heart health.

Yoga sequences for heart issues provide a targeted approach to improving cardiovascular health. You may take proactive efforts toward healing your heart and general well-being by introducing these sequences into your practice with care and attention. Always keep your health in mind, and get tailored advice from your healthcare expert.

Chapter 5: Nutrition and Lifestyle for a Healthy Heart

Good health is a valuable asset, and the health of your cardiovascular system is at the center of it (literally). Nutrition and lifestyle choices are critical to general health and the development of a strong, steady heartbeat.

Tips for a Heart-Healthy Diet

Maintaining a heart-healthy diet is one of the most important lifestyle decisions you can make to protect your cardiovascular health. It entails not just understanding which foods are good for your heart, but also developing behaviors that create a long-term, health-focused connection with your diet. In this in-depth investigation, we'll look into helpful hints for a heart-healthy diet and provide ten nutritious meals that adhere to these principles, packed with preparation directions and estimated prep times.

Dietary Guidelines for a Heart-Healthy Lifestyle

1. Support Whole Foods:

 - Fruits, vegetables, whole grains, legumes, nuts, and seeds are examples of unprocessed or minimally processed foods to include in your diet. These are high in vitamins, minerals, fiber, and antioxidants.

2. Mindful Portion Control:

 - Observe portion proportions to avoid overeating. Use smaller portions and pay attention to your body's hunger signals.

3. Limit Saturated and Trans Fats:

 - Limit your intake of foods high in saturated fats (found in red meat, full-fat dairy, and tropical oils) and trans fats (found often in processed and fried foods).

4. Select Healthy Fats:

 - Unsaturated fats, such as those found in olive oil, avocados, and fatty seafood like salmon, are good for your heart.

5. Prioritize Omega-3 Fatty Acids:

 - Include omega-3 foods in your diet, such as flaxseeds, walnuts, and fatty seafood. These fats help to decrease inflammation and promote heart health.

6. Include Fiber-Rich Foods:

 - Fiber-rich foods such as oats, legumes, and whole grains help decrease cholesterol and enhance digestive health.

7. Limit Sodium Intake:

 - Cutting back on salt in your diet will help you regulate your blood pressure. Choose low-sodium alternatives and season with herbs and spices.

8. Lean Protein Sources:

- Choose lean protein sources such as chicken, fish, tofu, and lentils. These include vital amino acids without a lot of saturated fat.

9. Reduce Sugar Consumption:

- Reduce your intake of added sugars, which are commonly found in sugary drinks, candies, and processed meals. Choose natural sweeteners such as honey or fresh fruit.

10. Hydrate Wisely:

- Water is necessary for good health. Reduce your intake of sugary beverages and caffeine, and prioritize water hydration.

10 Recipes for Heart Health

1. Salmon with Lemon-Dill Sauce:

- Method: Baked salmon fillets with a fresh lemon-dill sauce.

- Preparation time: 30 minutes.

2. Quinoa and Black Bean Salad:

- Method: A protein-rich salad made with quinoa, black beans, fresh vegetables, and a lime-cilantro dressing.

- Preparation time: 20 minutes.

3. Mediterranean Chickpea dish:

- Method: A substantial dish of chickpeas, cherry tomatoes, cucumbers, olives, and feta cheese drizzled with balsamic vinaigrette.

- Preparation time: 15 minutes.

4. Avocado and Spinach Smoothie:

- Method: A creamy, green smoothie with avocado, spinach, banana, Greek yogurt, and almond milk.

- Preparation time: 10 minutes.

5. Roasted Vegetable Quiche:

- Method: A delicious quiche stuffed with roasted veggies and topped with a whole wheat crust.

- Preparation time: 45 minutes.

6. Greek Salad with Grilled Chicken:

- Method: A traditional Greek salad with grilled chicken breasts and a lemon-oregano dressing.

- Preparation time: 25 minutes.

7. Walnut-Crusted cooked Cod:

- Method: Cod fillets cooked to perfection in a walnut crust.

- Preparation time: 30 minutes.

8. Spiced Lentil Soup:

- Method: A hearty soup made with lentils, tomatoes, and a fragrant spice combination.

- Preparation time: 40 minutes.

9. Berry and Yogurt Parfait:

- Method: Layered parfait with Greek yogurt, fresh berries, honey, and granola.

- Preparation time: 10 minutes.

10. Stuffed Bell Peppers:

- Method: Stuffed bell peppers with lean ground turkey, brown rice, black beans, and seasonings.

- Preparation Time: 50 minutes.

Incorporating these heart-healthy techniques and dishes into your diet not only feeds your cardiovascular system but also benefits your overall health. Keep in mind that eating a heart-healthy diet is a long-term commitment, and that tiny, sustainable improvements can result in considerable health advantages over time.

The Importance of Mindfulness in Eating

Mindfulness in Eating: Nourishing the Body and Soul

In our fast-paced environment, eating is frequently a hurried, thoughtless action. We eat on the move, multitask, and often hardly notice the flavor and texture of our food. This lack of attention in eating can have serious ramifications for our health, particularly our heart health. In this investigation, we'll look at the importance of mindfulness in eating, its relationship to heart health, and practical ways to incorporate it into your everyday life.

The Mind-Body Connection

In the field of health, the heart-mind link is a well-established idea. It recognizes the close link that exists between our emotional and mental well-being and the health of our cardiovascular system. Stress, worry, and emotional turmoil can all contribute to poor eating habits, excessive intake of harmful foods, and irregular blood pressure readings.

Mindful eating is a discipline that connects heart health with mental well-being. It promotes mindful, in-the-moment awareness of what and how you consume. When you eat consciously, you do the following:

1. *Savor the Flavors*: You take the time to enjoy the flavor, texture, and scent of your meal, resulting in a more enjoyable eating experience.

2. *Recognize Hunger and Fullness:* Mindful eating allows you to tune into your body's hunger and fullness cues, which helps you avoid overeating.

3. *Minimize Stress*: Being in the now can help to minimize stress and emotional eating.

4. *Improve Digestion:* Mindful eating improves improved digestion by enabling your body to concentrate on the activity at hand.

5. *Increase Food Choices:* When you are conscious of what you eat, you are more likely to select nutritious food choices that are good for your heart.

Practical Mindful Eating Steps

1. *Eat Without Distractions:* Turn off electronics, put books and work away, and designate a separate area for eating.

2. *Chew Thoroughly:* Take your time with each bite, savoring the flavors and textures.

3. *Pause Between Bite:* Place your utensils down between bites to allow yourself time to taste the food and register sensations of fullness.

4. *Activate Your Senses:* Pay attention to the colors, scents, and textures of your meal. Involve all of your senses in the experience of eating.

5. *Listen to Your Body:* Be aware of hunger and fullness signals. Eat only when you're hungry and quit when you're full.

6. *Express Gratitude:* Take a few moments to thank your food. Consider where it comes from and the effort that went into making it.

7. *Slow Down:* Eating slowly encourages your body to convey fullness signals to your brain, lowering your chances of overeating.

8. *Regular Practice:* Mindful eating is a skill that develops with repetition. Be gentle with yourself as you establish this habit.

Heart Health and Mindful Eating

Mindful eating can improve heart health by lowering stress, assisting with weight control, and promoting healthier food choices. We are less prone to turn to comfort eating or consume excessive amounts of harmful foods when we eat thoughtfully.

If you include mindfulness into your eating habits, you will not only fuel your body but also your emotional and mental well-being. It's a simple yet powerful technique that promotes heart-mind balance.

Lifestyle Choices for Cardiovascular Wellness

Our hearts, the rhythmic powerhouses that keep us alive, demand our undivided attention and care. However, amid the rush and bustle of modern life, we frequently ignore the importance of lifestyle choices in promoting cardiovascular health. A heart-healthy lifestyle is more than just avoiding bad behaviors; it is a comprehensive commitment to making everyday decisions that emphasize the health of our hearts.

Comprehensive Cardiovascular Wellness

Cardiovascular wellness includes more than simply physical heart health. It includes emotional, mental, and social well-being. It's about taking a holistic approach that understands the interdependence of various aspects of life and how they affect the heart's health collectively.

Heart-Healthy Nutrition

Good nutrition is the bedrock of cardiovascular health. A heart-healthy diet includes plenty of fruits and vegetables, whole grains, lean meats, and healthy fats. It's all about filling your dish with bright colors and nutritious ingredients.

Consider John, a patient of mine who wanted to take care of his heart health through food. He recognized the nutritional value of fruits and vegetables, adding a rainbow of food into his meals. He began his day with a substantial dish of porridge sprinkled with fresh berries and heart-healthy walnuts.

John also made a point of eating lean proteins like grilled salmon or skinless chicken breast, as well as plant-based proteins like lentils and tofu. He preferred olive oil for cooking and sprinkling over salads, appreciating the flavor as well as the health advantages of monounsaturated fats.

John's experience demonstrates the transformative potential of mindful eating. He started eating in smaller portions, savoring each meal, and responding to his body's hunger and fullness cues. His heart-healthy decisions not only enhanced his physical health but also fed his spirit over time.

Physical Activity: A Passion for Movement

Another important component of cardiovascular fitness is regular physical activity like yoga. It helps to strengthen the heart muscle, enhance circulation, regulate weight, decrease inflammation, and reduce stress. Exercise, in all of its forms, is a love affair with movement that pays off handsomely for the heart.

Sarah, a mid-fifties patient, accepted this fact. She found her love of yoga and wanted to include it into her daily routine. The trails were her haven, where she could not only test her physically but also find consolation for her spirit. The rhythm of her asanas and the beauty of nature's breathing filled her heart with joy.

Sarah's dedication to her yoga program improved her cardiovascular health over time. Her resting heart rate dropped, her blood pressure level remained stable, and her general fitness increased.

Stress Reduction: A Breath of Fresh Air

Chronic stress can be harmful to our hearts. As a result, stress management is an essential component of cardiovascular wellbeing. Meditation, yoga, deep breathing, and mindfulness are not frills; they are critical components of our heart-healthy armory.

Consider the case of Michael, a corporate executive who was no stranger to the high-pressure demands of his profession. Mindfulness meditation provided him with solace. He set aside time each morning to sit quietly, focusing on his breath and establishing a sense of peace despite the commotion.

Michael's heart began to profit from this simple yet deep exercise as the weeks progressed into months. His blood pressure returned to normal, and he felt himself more prepared to manage the rigors of his job. Michael's experience demonstrates the transforming impact of stress management for cardiovascular wellbeing.

Quality Sleep: The Rejuvenating Embrace of the Heart

Quality sleep is an often-overlooked component of cardiovascular health. Sleep deprivation can cause a variety of health problems, including an increased risk of heart disease. Prioritizing sleep and sticking to a consistent sleep pattern is a self-care practice that the heart profoundly values.

Consider Emma's story as a young mother of two. Motherhood's duties frequently left her sleep-deprived, affecting her attitude and overall well-being. Emma resolved to prioritize sleep in her life. She created a distraction-free sleep environment by establishing a relaxing nighttime ritual.

Emma's sleep quality increased with time, and her energy levels skyrocketed. Her heart rejoiced in the revitalizing embrace of sound slumber. Her tale demonstrates the critical importance of good sleep for cardiovascular health.

Smoking Cessation, Alcohol Moderation, and Social Connections

Avoiding smoking and drinking in moderation are important lifestyle decisions for heart health. Tobacco use is a major risk factor for heart disease, and excessive alcohol use can be harmful to the heart. Smoking cessation and moderate alcohol use are deeds of love for your heart.

Social ties are also important for cardiovascular health. Strong connections and social bonds can help to alleviate stress and improve emotional well-being.

Lifelong Learning and Consistent Monitoring

Regular check-ups with your doctor are vital for maintaining your heart health. These examinations allow for the early diagnosis of risk factors and the development of individualized measures for heart disease prevention. Your healthcare team may advise you on lifestyle choices that are specific to your requirements.

Another part of cardiovascular fitness is lifelong learning and mental stimulation. Reading, puzzles, and learning new skills are all activities that challenge and excite your brain and are related with better heart health.

It is not a difficult undertaking to incorporate these lifestyle choices into your everyday life; it is an act of self-love and empowerment. Cardiovascular wellbeing is an ongoing journey of self-discovery and self-care. It's about appreciating your heart for its significance in your total well-being, not simply for its physical function.

Keep in mind that your heart is the center of your being. You empower yourself to live a meaningful, vibrant life by prioritizing its health. Each pulse is an encouragement to embrace a heart-healthy lifestyle that acknowledges the amazing organ that keeps you alive.

The decisions you make today will be echoed in the rhythm of your heart the next day. Choose wisely, take care of your cardiovascular health, and start on a journey filled with energy, resilience, and joy—a path that recognizes the heart as more than just a physical organ, but as the very essence of your existence.

Chapter 6: Yoga for Specific Heart Conditions

Yoga for Hypertension (High Blood Pressure)

High blood pressure, also known as hypertension, is known as the "silent killer" because it can harm your cardiovascular system without causing symptoms. If neglected, it can lead to major health problems such as heart disease and stroke. While medication therapies are necessary, including yoga into your hypertension control regimen can be a game changer for your heart health.

How to Understand Hypertension

Before getting into yoga's therapeutic power, it's important to understand hypertension. It happens when the force of the blood on the arterial walls is consistently too strong. This pressure on the arteries might cause them to become less elastic and more prone to blockages over time. Yoga takes a comprehensive approach to reducing high blood pressure, addressing both the physical and mental aspects that contribute to it.

Yoga Relationship

Yoga is a profound mind-body practice steeped in ancient knowledge, not merely physical postures. Yoga can help relieve stress, enhance circulation, and promote relaxation via conscious breathing, gentle movement, and meditation. These are all important aspects of hypertension management.

<u>Yoga Poses for High Blood Pressure</u>

Here are a few yoga positions that are very good for those who have high blood pressure:

1. Savasana (Corpse stance): This is a relaxing stance. By resting flat on your back with your arms and legs outstretched, you enable your body to relax and your mind to quiet.

2. Adho Mukha Svanasana (Downward-Facing Dog): This mild inversion position stretches and strengthens the whole body while increasing blood flow to the brain.

3. Viparita Karani (Legs Up the Wall Pose): You lift your legs against a wall in this restorative position. It induces relaxation and can aid in blood pressure reduction.

4. Bhujangasana (Cobra Pose): Cobra stretches the spine while strengthening the abdominal muscles. It has the potential to boost the circulatory system.

5. Anulom Vilom Pranayama (Alternate Nostril Breathing): In this breathing method, you inhale and exhale via alternating nostrils. It aids in the equilibrium of the neurological system and the reduction of stress.

The Mind-Body Relationship

Yoga's capacity to integrate the mind and body is one of its most profound qualities. Stress is a common contributor to hypertension. Yoga, via mindfulness and meditation, provides a way to deal with stress. By using these tactics on a daily basis, you may limit the production of stress hormones, which will help lower your blood pressure.

The Value of Consistency

Yoga for hypertension advantages, like any therapy, become more evident with persistent practice. Yoga should be included into your everyday practice, or at least multiple times each week. It's not about being a yoga guru; it's about using yoga to manage your hypertension and improve your general well-being.

Seek the advice of your healthcare provider

It is critical to contact with your healthcare physician before beginning any new fitness or wellness program, especially if you have a medical condition such as hypertension. They can provide you tailored advice on how to include yoga into your hypertension control regimen.

Yoga for high blood pressure is a path of self-discovery and self-care. It's a road that leads to improved heart health as well as enhanced inner serenity and well-being. Yoga practice can help you develop a stronger connection between your mind and body, leading to a healthier heart and a more vibrant existence.

Yoga for Stress-Related Heart Conditions

Heart disease, a fierce foe to health and vigor, claims millions of lives worldwide. Medical science provides critical interventions, including as drugs and surgery, to battle this illness and promote recovery. However, in our search for healing, we must not underestimate yoga's tremendous influence on heart health, particularly in the context of cardiac rehabilitation and other heart-related diseases. Stress, a terrible modern ailment, has serious consequences for heart health. Chronic stress has a role in the development and worsening of heart-related diseases such as hypertension, atherosclerosis, and arrhythmias. As we traverse the choppy seas of our everyday life, the ancient practice of yoga emerges as a beacon of hope, providing respite for the restless mind and healing for the troubled heart.

Understanding Stress and Its Relationship to the Heart

Before we go into the transforming realm of yoga, we must first understand the complex link between stress and heart health. Chronic stress triggers a series of physiological reactions, including the release of stress hormones such as cortisol and adrenaline. These hormonal surges wear on the cardiovascular system over time, causing high blood pressure, inflammation, and the formation of arterial plaque.

Stress also has a negative impact on heart health via behavioral mechanisms. Stress can lead to poor coping techniques such as overeating, smoking, or excessive alcohol use, which increases the risk of heart disease.

Yoga: An Ancient Stress-Relieving Technique

Yoga, a comprehensive method that unites the mind, body, and spirit, offers a respite from the contemporary world's never-ending demands. Here's how it can benefit those with stress-related cardiac conditions:

1. Stress Reduction: At the basis of yoga lies mindfulness— a mental state of focused awareness that anchors us in the present moment. Mindfulness meditation, a major component of yoga, helps the mind to stay calm and

focused in the midst of life's storms. This technique not only reduces stress but also decreases blood pressure and improves heart rate variability, all of which are indicators of cardiac health.

2. Physical Relaxation: By releasing muscle tension, yoga asanas (poses) promote physical relaxation. Poses such as Savasana (Corpse Pose) and Balasana (Child's Pose) are very helpful at inducing a state of profound relaxation, which is beneficial to the heart.

3. Controlled Breathing: Pranayama, or yogic breath control, is essential for nervous system relaxation. Techniques such as diaphragmatic breathing and alternative nostril breathing can help you manage stress-related cardiac issues.

4. Improved Cardiovascular Function: Inversions like Viparita Karani (Legs Up the Wall Pose) and heart-opening positions like Ustrasana (Camel Pose) improve blood circulation, which is crucial for cardiovascular health.

5. Lifestyle Change: Yoga promotes a comprehensive well-being approach. Practitioners are urged to live better lifestyles, such as mindful eating, frequent exercise, and supportive relationships—choices that are critical for stress management and heart health.

MBSR (Mindfulness-Based Stress Reduction)

The Mindfulness-Based Stress Reduction (MBSR) program is one notable use of yoga in stress-related cardiac problems. Dr. Jon Kabat-Zinn developed MBSR, which blends mindfulness meditation and yoga to manage stress-related health conditions such as heart disease. Numerous studies have shown that it can reduce stress, improve mental well-being, and improve heart health.

Consultation and Safety;

While yoga has a variety of advantages for stress-related cardiac diseases, it is critical to proceed with caution and under the supervision of a healthcare expert. Individuals with cardiac issues should see their doctor before beginning a yoga practice. They should also practice with a certified yoga instructor who has expertise customizing yoga for cardiac patients.

Finally, yoga is a light of hope for people suffering from stress-related cardiac diseases. It not only soothes the restless mind, but it also heals the troubled heart. Individuals who practice yoga as a stress-management technique can start on a path toward inner peace and heart health, allowing them to overcome life's problems with grace and ease.

Chapter 7: Yoga and Meditation for Emotional Well-Being

Yoga and meditation together open the path to great well-being. Yoga nourishes the body, meditation calms the mind, and the two work together to produce an inner symphony. This brief introduction provides an overview of the transforming potential of these ancient practices when combined, laying the groundwork for a more in-depth examination of their extraordinary benefits.

The Heart-Mind Connection

The heart, regarded as the physical organ responsible for life, also plays a symbolic function that is firmly established in our language and society. We talk about sincere sentiments, wear our hearts on our sleeves, and characterize love as something that comes from the heart. However, research has shown a significant link between the heart and the mind, a symbiotic interaction that shapes not just our emotional experiences but also our general health and well-being.

The Physiology of the Heart-Mind Connection

The autonomic nervous system, a complex network of nerves that governs involuntary physiological activities, is at the heart of this link. It is divided into two parts: the sympathetic nervous system (also known as the "fight or flight" system) and the parasympathetic nervous system (also known as the "rest and digest" system). These systems collaborate to preserve physiological homeostasis.

Both branches have an effect on the heart, which is a critical organ. During times of stress or excitement, the sympathetic nervous system urges the heart to beat faster and with more energy, preparing the body for action. The parasympathetic nervous system, on the other hand, decreases the heart rate, facilitating rest and healing.

The Heart and Emotional Intelligence

Emotions are important in the heart-mind link. Through a complicated network of neurons and chemicals, the heart interacts with the brain, impacting our emotional experiences. Emotions have been proven in studies to impact heart rate variability, which is a measure of the heart's capacity to adjust to changing situations. Positive emotions, such as pleasure and appreciation, are related with greater heart rate variability, which is suggestive of excellent heart health.

HRV (Heart Rate Variability)

HRV is a measure of the equilibrium of the sympathetic and parasympathetic neural systems. It is a key sign of cardiovascular health as well as mental well-being. High HRV levels are associated with improved stress resilience, emotional modulation, and overall heart health.

The Effects of Chronic Stress

Chronic stress, on the other hand, which is a feature of modern life, can disrupt the heart-mind link. Prolonged stress activates the sympathetic nervous system, causing an increase in heart rate and blood pressure. This can lead to heart disease and other health problems over time.

Mindfulness and Heart-Mind Integration

Meditation and deep breathing, for example, emerge as effective methods for developing the heart-mind link. They activate the parasympathetic nervous system, facilitating relaxation and stress reduction. Mindfulness meditation has been demonstrated to boost HRV while also improving emotional well-being and heart health.

The Importance of Love and Social Relationships

Love, which is frequently connected with concerns of the heart, is also important in the heart-mind relationship. Positive social relationships and professions of love stimulate the production of hormones such as oxytocin, which promote emotional well-being and cardiovascular health. Strong social support is associated with a lower risk of heart disease and living a longer, healthier life.

Finally, the heart-mind link demonstrates the complicated interplay between our emotions, physiology, and general well-being. We may boost both emotional and cardiovascular health by nourishing this relationship via techniques such as mindfulness, establishing strong social interactions, and controlling stress. It serves as a reminder that the heart is more than simply a physical organ; it is also a source of our innermost emotions and a key to our health and longevity. Accepting the fundamental heart-mind link sets you on a path to a better, happier existence.

Heart-Centered Meditation Practices

Meditation, or the practice of quieting the mind and focusing within, is a powerful doorway to emotional well-being and heart health. There is a unique kind of meditation called as heart-centered practices. These practices are intended to promote pleasant emotions, increase compassion, and nourish the heart, which is at the heart of our emotional experiences.

The Emotional Compass of the Heart

The heart has long been thought to be the core of our emotional experiences. We link this essential organ with sentiments of love, compassion, appreciation, and empathy. And scientific evidence suggests that our emotions have a significant influence on our general well-being, particularly our heart health.

Definition of Heart-Centered Meditation

Heart-centered meditation is a technique that focuses our attention and purpose on the heart region, promoting emotional balance and eliciting happy emotions. It boils down to opening one's heart and radiating love, kindness, and compassion—first to oneself, then to others.

Practices of Heart-Centered Meditation

1. Metta (Loving-Kindness Meditation): This exercise entails quietly repeating statements such as "May I/you be happy, healthy, and live with ease." We nurture sentiments of love and compassion by spreading these well-wishes to ourselves, loved ones, acquaintances, and even people with whom we disagree.

2. Heartfulness Meditation: In this approach, we concentrate our attention on the heart area and imagine a brilliant light or a sensation of warmth and love extending from the heart. This technique can elicit intense sensations of love and appreciation.

3. Compassion Meditation (Karuna): Compassion meditation, like loving-kindness meditation, directs our kind desires toward people who are suffering. We may improve our own well-being and the well-being of others by nurturing sentiments of empathy and compassion.

4. Gratitude Meditation: This technique entails thinking on the things in our lives for which we are grateful. We open our hearts to pleasant feelings by recognizing our benefits and expressing thanks.

5. Heart Chakra Meditation: This meditation, based on ancient yogic traditions, focuses on the heart chakra, an energy center connected with love and compassion. This energy area is activated and balanced via visualizations and affirmations.

The Science of Heart-Centered Meditation

According to research, heart-centered meditation practices can have a significant impact on our emotional and physical well-being. They alleviate stress, lower blood pressure, increase heart rate variability, and promote emotional resilience. These routines help strengthen sentiments of connection with others and improve our ability for empathy and compassion.

How to Implement Heart-Centered Meditation in Your Life;

You don't have to be a seasoned meditator to reap the advantages of heart-centered meditation. Beginners might begin with short sessions and progressively increase their practice time. A few minutes of heart-centered meditation each day can result in considerable improvements in emotional well-being and cardiovascular health.

Finally, heart-centered meditation techniques provide a transforming path to emotional well-being and heart health. We not only improve our own lives by cultivating good emotions, encouraging compassion, and opening our hearts, but we also contribute to a world were love and kindness reign supreme. If you embrace these practices, you will be on your way to a more compassionate, joyous, and heart-centered living.

Yoga Can Help You Develop Emotional Resilience

The value of emotional resilience cannot be emphasized in today's fast-paced and frequently stressful world. Emotional resilience is the ability to adapt to and recover from adversity, stress, and the unavoidable setbacks of life. It's a trait that allows people to negotiate the ebb and flow of emotions, promoting mental health. While there are several techniques for improving emotional resilience, one increasingly acknowledged and successful option is yoga practice.

Yoga, an ancient Indian discipline, is highly praised for its numerous advantages that include physical, mental, and spiritual well-being. A complex tapestry of approaches targeted at fostering emotional resilience exists in addition to the physical postures, or asanas, that people identify with yoga. Yoga offers a comprehensive arsenal for anyone wishing to strengthen their emotional well-being, ranging from mindful breathing to meditation and heart-centered practices.

The Mind-Body Connection: Understanding Yoga's Emotional Impact

The recognition of the fundamental link between the mind and the body is central to yoga's efficacy in fostering emotional resilience. The yogic philosophy understands the deep relationship between emotional well-being and physical health. Practitioners not only improve their bodies but also build mental fortitude by participating in physical postures, breathwork, and meditation.

Emotional Release Through Physical Postures

Asana practice entails deliberate movements and postures that enhance flexibility, strength, and balance. However, the advantages go beyond the physical realm. Many yoga poses are intended to relieve tension held in certain parts of the body, which is frequently related with mental stress. Heart-opening postures like as Camel Pose and Bridge Pose, for example, are said to relieve emotional blockages trapped in the chest, encouraging a sense of openness and vulnerability that can lead to emotional resilience.

Emotional Regulation and Breathing

Pranayama, or conscious breath control, is a key part of yoga. Various breathing techniques can produce relaxation, regulate the neurological system, and reduce stress. Practitioners gain an awareness of the influence of their breath on their emotional state through focused and deliberate breathing. This increased awareness becomes a crucial tool in controlling emotions, especially during difficult times.

Emotional Awareness Meditation

Meditation is an important component of many yoga practices, and it has tremendous advantages for emotional resiliency. Meditation, by building mindfulness and present-moment awareness, enables people to notice their thoughts and emotions without getting overwhelmed by them. This improved self-awareness builds the framework for better emotional reactions and a higher ability to deal with life's ups and downs.

Success Story: David's Journey to Emotional Resilience Through Yoga

David's tale exemplifies yoga's transforming effect in creating emotional resilience. David, a high-achieving professional with a demanding career, was experiencing increased stress, worry, and emotional tiredness. The continual strain of deadlines and expectations wore on his mental health, impacting not just his profession but also his relationships and entire quality of life.

David chose to try yoga to gain balance and emotional stability because he felt motivated to make a positive change. He went to his first yoga session with an open mind, despite his initial skepticism. Physical posture practice tested him both cognitively and physically, but it was the combination of breathwork and meditation that truly spoke to David.

David realized the powerful influence of yoga on his emotional landscape via persistent practice. Yoga poses gave a physical outlet for the accumulated stress in his body, giving a sensation of lightness and comfort. He was able to negotiate stressful situations with increased calm and clarity because to the careful breathwork.

During a meditation retreat aimed at fostering emotional resilience, David's journey took a significant turn. He dived into practices geared at identifying and processing emotions without judgment, guided by an experienced yoga instructor. This life-changing experience taught David to accept vulnerability and find greater strength in the face of hardship.

David saw a significant improvement in his emotional well-being over time. He grew less reactive to stresses, instead displaying greater toughness and flexibility. His connections improved as he developed a greater empathy and understanding for himself and others. The good changes were obvious not just by David, but also by people around him, who commented on his newfound feeling of peace and emotional equilibrium.

David's success story demonstrates how yoga may act as a trigger for emotional resilience. His experience exemplifies the transforming power of yoga, which provides a comprehensive approach to well-being that goes beyond the physical and into the depths of emotional and mental strength.

Integrating Yoga into Your Emotional Resilience Journey

David's story demonstrates that cultivating emotional resilience via yoga is a personal and ever-changing journey. Whether you are a seasoned yogi or a novice, the objective is to practice consistently and mindfully. Here are some simple actions you may take to incorporate yoga into your life for improved emotional well-being:

1. Begin with a Beginner-Friendly Class: If you're new to yoga, try enrolling in a beginner-friendly class or using online instructions. Concentrate on fundamental postures first, then progress to more complex activities.

2. Investigate Breathing methods: Start implementing easy pranayama methods into your regular practice. Deep belly breathing and alternate nostril breathing can both help to relax the nervous system.

3. Incorporate Mindfulness Meditation: Make time for mindfulness meditation. Begin with short sessions and progressively increase the time as you gain confidence in the practice. There are several guided meditations accessible online to help you on your path.

4. Include Heart-Opening positions in Your Practice: Include heart-opening yoga positions in your practice. These postures, such as Cobra or Fish, can help relieve chest tension and increase emotional openness.

5. Attend Yoga seminars or Retreats: Attend seminars or retreats that emphasize emotional resilience and mindfulness. These immersive experiences can help you to enhance your practice and get useful insights on emotion management.

Chapter 8: Your Heart-Healthy Yoga Journey

The book's last chapter, "Your Heart-Healthy Yoga Journey," leads readers on a personalized investigation of incorporating yoga into their life for cardiovascular fitness. This part stresses the development of a personalized yoga strategy, emphasizing the need of consistency and dedication. It encourages people to keep track of their development and to celebrate tiny triumphs along the road.

Furthermore, the chapter shares motivating success stories, establishing a sense of community and drive. The ultimate objective is to inspire readers to make a lifelong commitment to heart health by engaging in transformational yoga practices.

Creating a Personalized Yoga Plan

Developing a tailored yoga plan is an important step in reaping the full benefits of yoga for heart health and overall well-being. Yoga becomes a sustainable and pleasurable part of your daily routine when it is tailored to your unique requirements, tastes, and health considerations. This chapter will provide in-depth information on the components of creating a personalized yoga plan as well as a sample plan to help you on your way.

Understanding Your Needs and Objectives:

1. Physical Health Evaluation: Begin by evaluating your present physical health. Make a note of any existing medical issues, injuries, or limits. Consult a healthcare specialist to ensure that your yoga activities are appropriate for your health.

2. Establishing Objectives: Clearly state your objectives for implementing yoga into your life. Having defined objectives will assist adapt your approach, whether it's boosting cardiovascular health, lowering stress, increasing flexibility, or a mix of these.

Selecting the Best Yoga Style:

1. Hatha Yoga as a Foundation: If you're new to yoga or prefer a mild approach, Hatha yoga might be a good place to start. It emphasizes on fundamental postures, breathing methods, and relaxation techniques.

2. Vinyasa for Dynamic Flow: Vinyasa yoga is a fluid series of postures connected with breath if you appreciate movement and want a more dynamic practice. It increases muscle strength, flexibility, and cardiovascular endurance.

3. Restorative Yoga for Relaxation: Consider adding restorative yoga for stress reduction and deep relaxation. It consists of passive positions assisted by props that promote relaxation and renewal.

Structuring Your Yoga Routine:

1. Warm-Up and Breathwork: Begin by doing simple warm-up exercises to get your body ready for activity. To focus your attention and relax your nervous system, use breathwork such as deep belly breathing or alternate nostril breathing.

2. Cardiovascular Health Asanas: Include heart-opening positions like Cobra, Bridge, and Warrior poses. These

postures help improve circulation, strengthen the heart, and relieve chest stress.

3. Flexibility and Strength: Incorporate postures that improve flexibility and strength, promoting total physical well-being. Balance is promoted by poses like Tree Pose and Warrior II, while strength is built by Plank and Downward-Facing Dog.

4. Cool Down and Relaxation: Finish your practice with some relaxing positions and techniques. Savasana (Corpse Pose) should be included to let your body and mind to fully absorb the benefits of your practice.

Adapting to Your Schedule:

1. Consistency is Key: Aim for regular, consistent practice. Find a regimen that works for you, whether it's a 20-minute session in the morning or a lengthier practice on weekends.

2. Duration Flexibility: Your yoga approach should be adjustable to changing time limits. A shorter session might be just as effective as a longer one on a hectic day. Prioritize quality over quantity.

Paying Attention to Your Body:

1. Adjust Poses as Needed: Pay attention to your body's cues. If a position causes discomfort or agony, alter it or skip it. Yoga should be a source of nourishment rather than stress.

2. Go at Your Own Pace: Allow yourself to go at your own pace. If you're new to yoga, begin with basic positions and work your way up to more advanced practices as your strength and flexibility develop.

Personalized Yoga Plan Example:

Routine for the Morning (20 minutes):

- Warm-up (5 minutes): Neck and shoulder rolls, mild twists

- Sun Salutation A: (5 minutes) Flow through a series of positions connected with breath.

- Poses for Opening the Heart: Cobra Pose, Warrior I, Warrior II (5 minutes)

- Strength and Balance: Tree Pose, Plank, and Downward-Facing Dog (3 minutes)

- Relaxation: Forward fold, Child's Pose (2 minutes)

Evening Routine (30 minutes):

- Breathwork (5 minutes): alternate nostril breathing, deep belly breathing

- Restorative Poses: Bridge Pose with Support, Legs Up the Wall (10 minutes)

- Relaxation and Flexibility: Seated Forward Bend, Butterfly Pose, Savasana (10 minutes)

- Mindfulness Meditation (5 minutes): Concentrate on your breathing or use a guided meditation.

This 365 Day-plan includes a range of poses and routines to keep your routine interesting and varied. Adjust the time and intensity to your preference, and remember to listen to your body.

Day 1:

- Morning (20 minutes): Sun Salutation A, Warrior II, Tree Pose

- Evening (30 minutes): Alternate nostril breathing, Seated Forward Bend, Savasana

Day 2:

 - Morning (25 minutes): Sun Salutation A, Downward-Facing Dog, Warrior III

- Evening (30 minutes): Restorative Bridge Pose, Legs Up the Wall, Mindfulness Meditation

Day 3:

 - Morning (20 minutes): Sun Salutation A, Chair Pose, Cobra Pose

- Evening (35 minutes): Deep belly breathing, Butterfly Pose, Plank, Savasana

Day 4:

- Morning (25 minutes): Sun Salutation A, Warrior I, Triangle Pose

- Evening (30 minutes): Restorative Child's Pose, Cat-Cow Stretch, Guided Meditation

Day 5:

- Morning (20 minutes): Sun Salutation A, Camel Pose, Downward-Facing Dog

- Evening (35 minutes): alternate nostril breathing, forward fold, warrior II, and Savasana

Alternate between morning and evening exercises, including a variety of postures and techniques. Here's a rough rule of thumb for variety:

- Morning Routines: To get your day started, focus on energetic postures, sun salutations, and standing positions.

- Evening Routines: To unwind and prepare for a comfortable sleep, emphasize relaxation, restorative postures, and meditation.

Feel free to repeat various exercises according on your preferences and to add or alter postures as you gain confidence. Remember, the objective is to develop a long-term and pleasurable practice that improves your entire well-being.

Tracking Your Progress and Success Stories

The process of adopting yoga into your life for heart health and overall well-being is about more than just physical postures and breathwork; it is also about the transformational development you make along the way.

This chapter discusses the importance of measuring your progress and includes motivating success stories to help readers on their personal yoga journey. There are also practical ideas on how to successfully measure progress.

Understanding the Importance of Progress Monitoring:

Tracking your development in yoga is a useful tool for various reasons:

1. Growth Visibility: Tracking your practice on a regular basis lets you to notice concrete changes in flexibility, strength, and general well-being. It is a graphical depiction of your adventure.

2. Drive and Accountability: Seeing improvement may be a strong motivation. It promotes consistency and dedication by demonstrating the good results of your efforts.

3. Adaptation and Adjustment: Tracking allows you to detect problem areas. You may modify your practice depending on your findings, whether it's improving a difficult position or devoting extra time to relaxation.

4. Mind-Body Relationship: The monitoring process promotes a stronger bond between the mind and body. As

you become more aware of your physical and mental states, you will develop a better understanding of how your yoga practice affects your entire well-being.

Successful Case Studies of Clients:

1. Sarah's Path to Strength and Flexibility:

 - Sarah, a busy professional, struggled at first with consistency. She steadily enhanced her strength and flexibility by recording her progress and committing to a 20-minute morning exercise. Her triumph exemplifies the transforming power of little, sustained efforts.

2. Mark's Stress Reduction Techniques Using Breathwork:

- Mark, who works in a high-stress environment, included breathwork into his nighttime routine. He noted a considerable reduction in stress and improved sleep patterns while tracking his stress levels and sleep quality. Mark's tale demonstrates the effectiveness of focused breathing in stress management.

3. Emily's Emotional Resilience as a Result of Meditation:

- Emily, who was dealing with emotional issues, incorporated meditation into her yoga practice. Emily noticed increased emotional resilience and a more optimistic attitude after measuring her emotional state before and after meditation sessions. Her experience highlights the emotional advantages of practicing mindfulness activities.

4. James' Cardiovascular Health: James, who was diagnosed with hypertension, devised a tailored yoga regimen that emphasized heart-healthy postures and stress reduction. James saw a steady improvement in his

cardiovascular health by regularly checking his blood pressure and speaking with his healthcare physician. His success story emphasizes the need of integrating yoga with medical supervision for certain health concerns.

How to Keep Track of Your Progress:

1. Keep a Yoga Journal: Keep a diary to chronicle your daily or weekly practice. Take note of the length of time, exact positions, and any observations or reflections. This written document serves as a physical chronicle of your adventure.

2. Make Use of Technology:

- Use applications or internet platforms created to track yoga practice. Many applications include capabilities for keeping track of practices, establishing goals, and even giving guided routines.

3. Before-and-After Evaluations:

- Evaluate your flexibility, strength, and overall well-being on a regular basis. Take pictures or keep a journal of your starting talents and compare them to your growth over time. Visual analogies may be inspirational.

4. Pay Attention to Your Body:

- Take note of how you feel before, during, and after each practice. Improve your mobility, lessen your stress, and boost your energy levels. These subjective ratings give useful information.

5. Establish clear, quantifiable goals:

- Set clear, quantifiable goals for your yoga practice. Having defined targets helps you trace your journey more efficiently, whether it's holding a tough posture for a longer length or attaining a certain level of flexibility.

Progress tracking is a dynamic and individualized component of your yoga practice. It entails more than simply bodily changes; it also includes mental, emotional, and spiritual development. You empower yourself to make the most of your yoga practice and feel its transforming effects by adopting a focused and purposeful approach to progress monitoring.

Staying Committed to Lifelong Heart Health: A Comprehensive Exploration

"Staying committed to lifelong heart health" encompasses a powerful concept that goes beyond temporary happiness and into the domain of long-term vitality and longevity. This is not a one-time commitment, but rather a lifelong path marked by mindful decisions, holistic practices, and steadfast dedication to the health of the heart, the figurative and literal center of our existence. In this investigation, we will look at the significance of this commitment, the advantages it provides, and practical techniques for implementing it into our everyday lives.

How to Understand the Commitment:

At the heart of the commitment to lifelong heart health is the realization that our cardiovascular health is substantially impacted by our lifestyle choices rather than heredity or chance. This is an agreement with oneself, understanding the importance of the heart to overall health and resolving to prioritize its care for the rest of one's life.

The dedication is adopting a proactive mentality in which individuals become builders of their own heart health destiny. It is a path that recognizes the interdependence of physical, mental, and emotional well-being.

Instead of viewing health as a destination, it is viewed as a constant process, a continuous investment in the basis of a vigorous and meaningful life.

Benefits of Maintaining Lifelong Heart Health:

1. Longevity and Quality of Life:

- Example: Consider people who practice a heart-healthy lifestyle their entire lives. Research regularly shows that such people live longer lives, not just in terms of years, but also in terms of their capacity to enjoy an active and satisfying life well into their senior years.

2. Reduced Cardiovascular Disease Risk:

- Example: Commitment to heart health reduces the risk of cardiovascular disorders, such as heart attacks and strokes. Individuals may establish a protective shield around their cardiovascular system by eating a heart-healthy diet, exercising regularly, and controlling stress.

3. Increased Energy and Vitality:

Example: Imagine waking up every morning full of life and energy. A lifetime commitment to heart health promotes enhanced blood circulation, appropriate oxygen delivery to cells, and efficient heart function. This leads in increased energy and a general sense of well-being.

4. Mental and Emotional Health:

- Example: The heart-mind link is an important element of committing to lifelong heart health. According to research, those who prioritize heart health had reduced levels of stress, anxiety, and sadness. This mental and emotional well-being improves overall quality of life.

5. Financial Savings and Lower Medical Costs:

- Example: Consider the long-term financial implications of cardiac health. A lifetime commitment to heart health may result in lower healthcare expenses related to cardiovascular illnesses. Investing in preventative measures, such as frequent check-ups and a healthy lifestyle, can result in significant long-term savings.

6. Better Cognitive Function:

- Example: A lifetime commitment to heart health has been related to improved cognitive function and a lower risk of cognitive decline as people age. better blood flow and oxygen availability to the brain lead to better cognitive capacities such as memory and problem-solving abilities.

Practical Heart Health Strategies for Life:

1. Adopting a Heart-Healthy Diet:

- Example: Consume a mix of fruits and vegetables, healthy grains, and lean proteins. Limit your intake of saturated fats, trans fats, and salt. A heart-healthy diet supplies necessary nutrients while encouraging normal cholesterol and blood pressure levels.

2. Consistent Physical Activity:

- Example: Make it a habit to exercise on a regular basis. Aim for 150 minutes of moderate-intensity aerobic activity each week or 75 minutes of vigorous-intensity aerobic activity. Cardiovascular fitness is enhanced by activities such as vigorous walking, running, swimming, and cycling.

3. Stress Management Techniques:

- Example: Include stress-relieving activities in your everyday routine. Yoga, meditation, deep breathing exercises, and mindfulness are all good stress-reduction techniques. By treating stress, you can reduce a major risk factor for heart disease.

4. How to Maintain a Healthy Weight:

- Example: Aim for a body weight that is within the healthy range for your height. A healthy weight contributes to proper heart function, minimizes the load on the circulatory system, and lowers the risk of obesity-related illnesses.

5. Regular Health Check-Ups:

- Example: Make regular appointments with your healthcare practitioner. Monitoring blood pressure, cholesterol levels, and other critical indicators enables early diagnosis of possible problems, allowing for prompt intervention and preventive actions.

6. Avoiding Tobacco and Reducing Alcohol Consumption:

- Example: Commit to living a tobacco-free lifestyle. Tobacco use is a major risk factor for heart disease. If you do drink, do so in moderation. Excessive alcohol consumption can lead to high blood pressure and other cardiovascular problems.

7. Developing Healthy Relationships:

- Example: Recognize the importance of social ties in terms of heart health. Develop supportive connections, participate in pleasant social interactions, and put your emotional well-being first. Strong social bonds are linked to a lower risk of heart disease.

8. Continuous Learning and Adaptation:

Example: Keep up-to-date on the latest heart-health research and guidelines. Be willing to change your way of life in response to new discoveries. A desire to adapt, evolve, and welcome good changes is required for a lifelong commitment.

Staying dedicated to lifelong heart health is, in essence, a vow to oneself—an acknowledgment of the inherent importance of a healthy heart and its significant influence on one's whole lifestyle.

The advantages extend beyond physical health to mental clarity, emotional resilience, and general quality of life. It's a commitment that endures, producing a legacy of happiness that reverberates down the generations, a monument to the enduring power of a heart that is fostered, safeguarded, and honored. It's a chorus of thanks for the enduring strength that comes from a heart cared for with love and commitment.

Caring for the Heart:

We nurture the heart by engaging in practices that recognize its emotional depth and resilience. It's the gentle rhythm of self-care routines such as periods of calm, appreciation for the present moment, and acts of compassion aimed both within and outward.

When we prioritize nutrition, exercise, and mental well-being, we create an environment in which the heart may thrive, pounding not just in existence but also in vibrancy.

Protecting the Heart:

Protection becomes a spiritual obligation, a pledge to shelter the heart from the turmoil of modern existence. It entails making decisions that are beneficial to the heart's health, such as eating nutritious meals, embracing stress-reduction techniques, and avoiding harmful habits. We build the heart by watchful guardianship, allowing it to beat with power and elegance throughout the seasons of life.

Celebrating the Heart:

Celebration is the song that follows each heartbeat, a beautiful acknowledgement of the trip taken. It is the acknowledgement of accomplishments, the achievement of milestones, and the ongoing dedication to heart health. Each moment of joy is a success - a tribute to the heart's constant rhythm and the indomitable spirit that pulls us ahead.

The Symphony of Endurance:

We witness a symphony of endurance in the lasting force of a heart that is fostered, safeguarded, and praised. It's a song made up of everyday decisions, triumphs against hardship, and thanks for the life energy that flows through our veins. This enduring force is a witness to the connectivity of the mind, body, and soul, not simply a physical occurrence.

The steady pulse of the heart mirrors the resilience formed of care, the strength developed through protection, and the joy found in celebration. It becomes a metaphor for life, a reminder that by lovingly caring to our hearts, protecting their well-being, and celebrating their vitality, we may achieve great things.

We build a music that resounds across time, leaving a legacy of lasting health and well-being. When a heart is fostered, safeguarded, and acknowledged, it becomes an everlasting testament to a life lived in accordance with one's most fundamental essence. HEART LIVES MATTER!

Conclusion: Embrace the Power of Yoga for a Healthier Heart

The appeal to prioritize heart health is more relevant than ever in the maze of modern living, where the pulse of existence is often drowned out by the noise of demands and diversions. As we read through the pages of this book, we come to a turning point - the conclusion that invites us to accept the transformational potential of yoga for a healthier heart.

Thoughts on the Journey:

Our journey through the realms of heart health and yoga has been like a tapestry, with strands of insight, practice, and deep realizations weaved throughout. We have begun on a comprehensive journey, from uncovering the delicate physiology of the heart to delving into the depths of yogic philosophy. The voyage has been more than just an examination of postures and breath; it has been a pilgrimage to the heart's sanctity, both as a physical organ and as the metaphorical seat of our innermost emotions.

We've dived into the very essence of heart health in the chapters before this conclusion, revealing the symbiotic link between yoga and the cardiovascular system. We've analyzed the science underlying the practices, investigated the fundamental principles of yoga, and navigated through heart-healthy sequences. Beyond the postures and breathwork, the essential heartbeat of this trip is the awareness that yoga is a philosophy, a way of life, and a deep instrument for feeding our hearts in every aspect.

The Heart Is More Than Just Muscle:

As we wrap up our investigation, it's critical to look at the heart through a lens that goes beyond its physiological purpose as a muscle that pumps blood. The heart is the source of our emotions, the orchestrator of our experiences, and the link between mind and body. Yoga, with its holistic approach, teaches us to see the heart not in isolation, but as an intricate tapestry of our being.

The heart often takes the weight of stress, emotions, and the never-ending demands of modern existence. It becomes a mute witness to our lives' turmoil, repeating not only the physical strain but also the emotional echoes of our experiences. Yoga, as a powerful ally, enters this battlefield, providing a refuge for the heart to find comfort, strength, and regeneration. It is an opportunity to blend physical postures with awareness, compassion, and emotional resilience.

Yoga's Transformative Power:

Yoga, at its foundation, is a transformational technology. It is a spiritual science that asks us to remove the layers of worry, anxiety, and emotional baggage that have accumulated around our hearts. Yoga, through the alchemy of breath, movement, and awareness, becomes a catalyst for transformation – not just in the physical body, but also in the fabric of our lives.

Consider the scientifically proven advantages of yoga for heart health. Gentle stretching and posture strengthening improve circulation and help the cardiovascular system. Breathwork, a fundamental component of yoga practice, modulates the autonomic nervous system, lowering tension and increasing relaxation.

The combination of physical movement and breath produces a symphony that vibrates through the chambers of the heart, promoting not just physical resilience but also emotional and mental well-being.

Yoga's power resides in its flexibility to individual demands. It is not a one-size-fits-all prescription, but rather a toolset that allows each practitioner to personalize their approach to their own needs. Yoga provides a range of practices that may be woven into the fabric of everyday life, whether it's the soothing embrace of restorative positions for stress reduction or the energizing rush of sequences for cardiovascular health.

A Customized Journey:

As we end, it is critical to emphasize the importance of a particular yoga journey. The heart, with its own rhythm, demands a practice that is sensitive to its intricacies. Each person on their path to heart health is an artist creating their masterpiece, with yoga as the canvas and the heart as the vitality brushstroke.

We've uncovered the tools for creating this masterpiece chapter by chapter, from learning core yoga concepts to studying heart-healthy sequences. The path does not end with a set of fixed rules, but rather with a living, breathing practice that changes with each breath and heartbeat. It is an invitation to be the architect of your own well-being, constructing a practice that corresponds to your requirements, objectives, and heart rhythm.

Success Stories to Celebrate:

Throughout our journey, we have come across triumphant stories – people who have experienced miraculous breakthroughs as a result of combining devotion and yoga. Consider Sarah, who discovered strength and flexibility via consistency, or Mark, who learned to manage stress with breathwork. These stories are not unique instances, but rather testaments to the universal potential that exists inside each of us.

These success tales are more than just anecdotes; they are lighthouses illuminating the way to a healthier heart. They are living proof of the power of yoga's transformational force and devotion. They serve as lighthouses, demonstrating that the path to heart health is a collaborative one, with each success story adding to the collective symphony of well-being.

The Adventure Continues:

As we approach the end of this book, let it serve as a starting point for the trip into the future of lifelong heart health. Yoga's transformational power is not limited to the pages of this book; it manifests itself in lived experiences, everyday practices, and a dedication to nourishing the heart in every breath.

Beyond these words, the journey continues into the hallowed place of your yoga mat, the sanctuary of your breath, and the rhythm of your heart. It is a constant dialogue with your body, an investigation of your emotional environment, and a celebration of your inner life.

Allow the end of this book to be the beginning of a lifelong commitment — an invitation to weave the knowledge of yoga into the very fabric of your being.

Embracing the Inner Power:

Finally, accept your inner strength – the power to nurture, defend, and honor your heart. As a guiding light, yoga lights the route to a healthier heart, providing not just physical advantages but also a holistic approach to well-being.

It is a celebration of inner strength, an acknowledgment of the enduring force that flows through every heartbeat. The ability to embrace a healthy heart is a practical reality that is ready to unfurl with each deliberate breath, every mindful movement, and the dedication to a life enriched with yoga knowledge.

May the conclusion of this book be the prologue to a tale of heart health, penned by you, fostered by yoga, and celebrated in the brilliant hues of well-being, in the magnificent tapestry of your existence.

As you take your first step, may your heart beat in time with the rhythm of life, a tribute to the enduring power of a heart that is not merely alive, but genuinely alive — thriving, joyful, and pulsing with the energy of a life well-lived.

As you start on this path, may your heart serve as a blank canvas for the transformational brushstrokes of yoga to produce a work of art of health, energy, and pleasure.

Appendix A: Recommended Resources and Further Reading

Knowledge becomes a guiding force on your quest toward a healthier heart via the transforming power of yoga. This appendix is a carefully chosen collection of resources and supplementary reading materials to help you develop your understanding, refine your practice, and discover new insights regarding heart health and yoga philosophy.

Books:

1. The Heart of Yoga: Developing a Personal Practice by T.K.V. Desikachar

- A seminal work exploring the philosophy and principles of yoga, offering valuable insights for creating a personalized practice.

2. The Science of Yoga: The Risks and Rewards by William J. Broad

- Delve into the scientific aspects of yoga, understanding its benefits and potential risks, providing a balanced perspective on its impact on health.

3. Yoga Anatomy by Leslie Kaminoff and Amy Matthews

- Explore the anatomy of key yoga poses, gaining a deeper understanding of how each posture affects the body, including its impact on heart health.

Websites:

1. Yoga Journal (www.yogajournal.com)

- A comprehensive online resource featuring articles, videos, and guides on various aspects of yoga, including sequences tailored for heart health.

2. American Heart Association (www.heart.org)

- The official website of the American Heart Association provides a wealth of information on heart health, including guidelines for exercise and stress management.

3. The International Association of Yoga Therapists (www.iayt.org)

- Explore resources related to the therapeutic application of yoga. The website offers insights into how yoga can be used as a complementary approach to healthcare.

Videos:

1. Yoga With Adriene (www.youtube.com/user/yogawithadriene)

- Adriene Mishler's YouTube channel offers a variety of yoga practices suitable for all levels. Look for specific sequences related to heart health and overall well-being.

2. Gaia (www.gaia.com)

- Gaia is an online platform with a vast library of yoga videos, including classes focused on heart health, meditation, and holistic well-being.

Heart Health Organizations and Support:

1. World Heart Federation (www.world-heart-federation.org)

- An organization dedicated to leading the global fight against cardiovascular disease. Their website provides valuable insights into heart health and prevention.

2. Mayo Clinic - Heart Disease Section (www.mayoclinic.org/diseases-conditions/heart-disease)

- Explore the Mayo Clinic's resources on heart disease, including articles, guides, and videos offering medical perspectives on cardiovascular health.

Remember that the path to a healthier heart is a combination of education, practice, and constant investigation. These tools act as companions on your journey, providing a variety of viewpoints and useful insights. Whether you want to learn more about yoga philosophy, improve your postures, or learn about the newest heart health studies, these recommendations offer a rich tapestry of knowledge to help your continuous wellness journey.

Appendix B: Glossary of Yoga Terms

Beginning a yoga journey entail being acquainted with the complex tapestry of language that characterizes this ancient practice. This glossary will help you navigate the complex language of yoga by offering definitions and explanations for major phrases. Whether you're a seasoned practitioner or a beginner to the mat, learning this terminology will help you gain a better knowledge of the philosophy, anatomy, and other parts that make up the world of yoga.

Asana: Physical postures or poses practiced in yoga.

Pranayama: Breath control exercises in yoga, emphasizing conscious and intentional breathing techniques.

Vinyasa: A flowing sequence of yoga poses coordinated with the breath, often forming a dynamic and continuous movement.

Namaste: A traditional greeting or gesture of respect in which one bows with hands together, saying "Namaste" as an acknowledgment of the divine in oneself and others.

Chakra: Energy centers within the body, according to yogic philosophy, associated with different aspects of life and consciousness.

Mantra: A sacred sound, word, or phrase repeated during meditation or chanting to aid concentration and spiritual connection.

Om (Aum): A sacred sound and a spiritual icon in Indian religions, often chanted at the beginning or end of yoga sessions.

Drishti: A focused gaze or point of focus, commonly used during yoga poses to enhance concentration and balance.

Savasana: Corpse Pose, a relaxation posture where the practitioner lies flat on their back, typically at the end of a yoga session.

Yogi/Yogini: A male (yogi) or female (yogini) practitioner of yoga.

Mudra: Hand gestures or symbolic hand positions used in meditation and yoga to channel energy and enhance the flow of prana.

Prana: Life force or vital energy, believed to circulate within the body, influencing physical and mental well-being.

www.ingramcontent.com/pod-product-compliance
Lightning Source LLC
Chambersburg PA
CBHW070850260726
48661CB00004B/1332